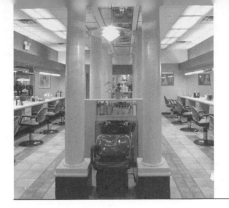

Milady's Successful Salon Management for Cosmetology Students

FIFTH EDITION

EDWARD J. TEZAK

MILADY

Australia • Canada • Mexico • ... ...ngdom • United States

D1145745

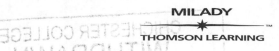

MILADY

™

THOMSON LEARNING

Successful Salon Management for Cosmetology Students
by Edward J. Tezak

MILADY STAFF:

President:
Susan L. Simpfenderfer

Publisher:
Marlene McHugh Pratt

Acquisitions Editor:
Pamela B. Lappies

Developmental Editor:
Judy Roberts

Executive Production Manager:
Wendy A. Troeger

Production Editor:
Eileen M. Clawson

Cover Design:
TDB Publishing Services

Executive Marketing Manager:
Donna J. Lewis

Channel Manager:
Wendy Mapstone

Text Design and Composition:
Publisher's Studio, a division of
Stratford Publishing Services

For permission to use material from this text or product, contact us by
Tel (800) 730-2214
Fax (800) 730-2215
www.thomsonrights.com

Library of Congress Cataloging-in-Publication Data
Tezak, Edward J.
    Successful salon management / Edward J. Tezak.—
5th ed.
        p. cm.
    New ed. of: Milady's salon management for
cosmetology students / Edward Tezak. 4th ed. 1993.
    Includes index.
    ISBN 1-56253-679-6
    1. Beauty shops—Management. I. Tezak, Edward J.
Milady's salon management for cosmetology students.
II. Title.
TT965.T493 2001
646.7'2'068—dc21   2001028138

NOTICE TO THE READER

Contents

CHAPTER SIX

Decorating and Arranging the Styling Area   65

CHAPTER SEVEN

The Supply Room   77

CHAPTER FIFTEEN

Key Points for Successful Salon Operation Reviewed   186

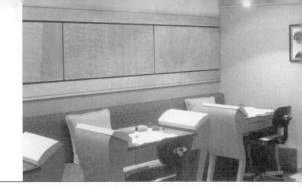

CHAPTER ONE

Salon Types and Their Locations

What Type of Salon Do You Want?

A number of salon types can be found in the beauty industry today. They can be broken down into four major groups, but there is constant overlapping between the groups. The four major groups of beauty salons are:

1. hotel
2. department store
3. shopping center
4. home-neighborhood salon

All beauty salons, regardless of how costly or modern their fixtures, will fit into one or more of these classes. Salons are found in shopping centers and home-neighborhood locations, but most large department stores have a salon, too. Skin-care areas are mostly found in large, full-service salons and department store salons.

Hotel Salons

Hotel salons are usually small operations. They consist of from two to eight operators. The space is leased by the hotel to the owner, who contracts to maintain an establishment in that hotel for a given number of years. Hotel customers have the convenience of a salon at their disposal without having to leave the premises. Unfortunately, the hotel usually does not have a sufficient amount of business to support the salon, so it must also serve the community at large in order to make a profit. Rent for this type of establishment will be slightly lower if the hotel feels that the beauty salon is an added service for its guests that will make them more likely to come back.

Contracts or lease agreements for hotel salons may contain certain unusual clauses, some of which are stated here.

1. Restrictions may be placed on where and what size sign you may use.
2. Cleaning and maintenance work may be provided by the hotel but charged to the owner in addition to the rent. In cases in which the establishment decides which cleaning firm does the maintenance work, be sure you know who has the right of supervision and control. There have been cases where the salon owner had no control of when the cleaning was to be done, how thorough it was, or how long the staff would work.
3. A charge system is sometimes in effect that allows hotel guests to charge beauty services on their overall hotel tab. In such cases, the hotel will make an adjustment with the salon in the form of a rent rebate or cash refund.
4. In some cases, hours during which the beauty salon is open or closed are regulated by the hotel.
5. Decorating can be a problem if there is a clause in the agreement giving the hotel the right to veto a salon decorating plan if they feel it will not go well with the other furnishings and decorations found in the hotel.

Should you wish to open a hotel salon, be sure you are clear about what is provided, what is expected, what the actual rent is, what hours the salon is to be open, and who has the responsibility for cleaning and maintenance.

Be sure of the bookkeeping system. Some hotels furnish their own bookkeeping service, while others let you select your own accountant. In case your rent is a percentage of yearly revenues, a time and place for yearly audit should be set up well in advance. This will enable you and your accountant to have sufficient time to gather all the information you need, thereby eliminating costly errors in your financial report.

Be sure that the contract with the hotel includes a procedure for handling dissatisfied clients. You must be in agreement about refund and redo policies.

Department Store Salons

The department store salon usually operates in a leased space. However, some department stores have recently opened their own salons. Major department stores usually contract with a nationwide chain of salons, and their operations can vary from a small salon to a multiunit salon of thirty to sixty operators. The chain makes its profit by mass purchasing and central supply depots. When a salon needs products, the home office is contacted, and the supplies are delivered. The supplies for this type of operation are usually ordered on a once-a-month basis, and each salon is well supplied with products. The waste in so ordering is offset by mass purchasing and special sales run at slow periods during the year to reduce over-stocked merchandise or dispose of products that are outdated.

All department store salons have certain things in common. The store usually supplies the accounting system and audit facilities. This is most convenient, as the store's charge system is always good in the beauty salon. The space in the store is usually rented or leased on a long-term contract, with a base rent and a percentage of sales after a certain gross figure is reached. An additional fee is charged for the cost of accounting and maintenance.

Some major factors to consider before owning or managing a department store salon are:

1. The image and clientele of the department store must be absolutely compatible with the image and clientele you want for the salon. The department store will draw clients for you; it does not work the other way around.
2. You need to know how much advertising the store will do during the year in their sales promotions. A store with a lot of traffic and a high gross sales figure will deliver more prospective customers to your salon than a store that is just keeping ahead of bankruptcy.
3. Who has the final word on complaints and adjustments that are part of day-to-day business? The store manager is much more likely than the salon manager to refund to a customer the money she paid for work she received, even though the work was of good quality. The store manager's reasoning may consider the fact that, while the store suffers the loss of the percentage of a salon service, the customer's good will may benefit the store in the long run. You may want to have more control over these situations, so definite rules should be set up for this in your contract.
4. Who will do the hair of clothes models hired for style shows? When should notice be given? What will be the charge or credit for this service? Answers

should be in your contract. In dealing with models, the hairstyle should be set by the salon's style director with the cooperation of the fashion show coordinator. Once a hairstyle is produced, it should not be changed or altered in any way. Consider the following case, in which a good deal of bad publicity was directed at the salon because of four teenage models who went home and rearranged their hairstyles before the start of the style show and looked amateurish. The programs merely read, "Hairstyle by _____ at the _____ salon." Compensation for styling models' hair should take the form of rent, advertising, or services and should appear on the books as some type of asset entry (cash received, rent, credit, advertising received, etc.).

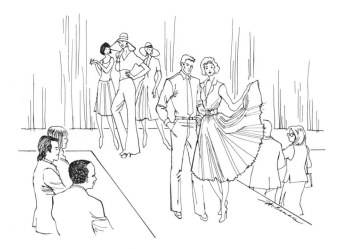

5. As with all business negotiations, such things as employee benefits, parking permits for employees, parking permits for customers, credit cards, accounting procedures, decoration coordination, advertising, and actual production time (store hours) should be clearly stated and fully understood by both the manager and the salon manager and/or owner.

Employees of a department store salon enjoy some important benefits that other salons do not offer: the use of a store lunchroom or cafeteria, employees' discount shopping, paid vacation, sick pay (sometimes), group insurance, and in some cases a profit-sharing program involving all store employees. The salon often has the advantage of national and local store-paid advertising of beauty products and salon services. As with all services and benefits offered to the employee, the salon must in some way carry its own share of the financial cost. As a result, the percentage to the operator of gross sales usually runs from 40 to 50 percent.

Salons in department stores are excellent places for skin- and nail-care services. A few problems should be considered, the most important of which relate to product sales and insurance.

1. Product sales. When the cosmetic area of the store sells the same skin- or nail-care products as the salon in the store, the products must be priced the same. The credit of the sale should go to the clerk or operator who sold the product. A problem arises, however, when the customer purchases the product at the cosmetic counter and wants the esthetician or manicurist to apply it at a reduced service fee. This is especially true in the nail technology and esthetician's service areas, where most of the charge to the client is to cover the salary of the operator and use of the equipment. A set policy should be established to handle this problem before it occurs.

2. Insurance. Certain cosmetics and nail-care products may cause skin reactions followed by the threat of lawsuits. Your contract should clearly spell out whose insurance pays the bill in case a judgment is reached: the department store, the salon, the operator, the cosmetic manufacturer, or a combination of all parties concerned? Since laws vary from state to state and new court cases set standards as the basis for judgments, the services of a good legal counselor is recommended before entering any contract in the salon business.

Shopping Center Salons

Like the corner grocer, the corner beauty salon has moved to larger quarters with ample parking for clients. Here they can serve a larger number of clients and offer a larger range of services. The size of this type of salon will vary; it usually has from two to eight operators. But, depending on the size of the center, it may contain more.

The rent is determined by a leasing agreement and may involve a flat rent plus a percentage figure after a certain level of gross sales is reached. This percentage of gross sales sometimes varies according to the length of time the shopping center has been in operation but usually is between 8 and 15 percent. A new approach is being tried, involving a decreasing percentage as the gross increases. This gives an added incentive for the salon owner to improve, increase, and expand. The base, or flat, rent is figured on a square foot per year basis. For example, a salon 30 feet by 70 feet has 2,100 square feet. At $10 a square foot, the annual base rent is $21,000 a year, or $1,750 a month.

Shopping centers usually operate on a multiyear lease with a cost of operation clause. This allows the rent to increase or decrease as the economy of the community changes due to inflation or depression. This enables the landlord to raise or lower the rent and the price of certain services without suffering any major loss of profit from investment.

Rents can vary greatly depending on the location, the type of mall, and the state of the economy, and you may be charged a percentage of your rent or space cost for mall upkeep, especially in an enclosed mall. Before deciding on a mall location, remember that all malls are not created equal. Like department stores, malls may have an orientation toward a particular type of shopper, for example, price-conscious as opposed to quality-conscious, or young and trendy as opposed to older and more classically conservative. And, while a strip mall does not give you the guaranteed traffic found in an enclosed mall, being stuck at the end of a little-traveled extension in an enclosed mall would put you out of the mainstream and would definitely affect your walk-in business.

The best way to handle negotiations for rent and other costs in such a mall is to know the location very well: demographics, traffic patterns, seasonal considerations, etc. Then hire an attorney or business consultant familiar with such negotiations to help you through the process. This will speed up the process and give you the best assurance of getting the best deal possible for yourself.

In a mall, an association of all shop owners is usually formed. The association dues are one major difference between a private, homeowner salon and a shopping center salon. Each usually owns his own business and has his own problems. The association helps to solve the common problems of doing business, such as snow removal, liability insurance, parking lot lighting, trash collection, and sometimes window washing. The association affords the individual shopkeeper a cooperative advertising program, in which the entire center will run a full-page ad as a sales promotion three or four times a year. Christmas decoration for the center can be coordinated by this association, and mutual landlord problems can be effectively handled.

When a shopping center opens, the landlord usually provides space for a beauty salon. This space is contracted for by square footage. It should be large enough for expansion but small enough to operate profitably. Some of the things a landlord will usually furnish are:

1. A floor (usually made of cement suitable for covering with tile, carpet, or wood).
2. Four walls (usually prepared for painting and with enough strength to support salon fixtures). The support construction tolerance and blueprint of your equipment installation should be analyzed prior to lease signing.
3. A ceiling (this is usually left rough but suitable to house a drop tile ceiling).
4. Some type of toilet facility (usually a toilet and sink left exposed).
5. A heater that will heat one large room (no ductwork).
6. Electrical connections to the area (no wiring work). Usually one light and a drop cord.
7. A display window and a door for customer service. A back door is usually provided.

Note: All of the preceding provisions are regulated by the state and the county in which you live. Check your local laws, rules, and regulations.

Whether or not we like shopping centers, they are here to stay. It has been stated that most consumer shopping, for both goods and services, will be in shopping centers in the future.

Home-Neighborhood Salons

The home-neighborhood salon is the oldest type of salon that still exists today. This form of salon can vary slightly:

1. The salon corporation or partnership owns the property and a residence, which is often connected to it. With this arrangement, the salon becomes more valuable day by day as the rent, which would otherwise be paid out, is used to pay for the purchase of the land and the building. The salon is worth the price of the equipment, the price of supplies on hand, investment for utilities (electrical wiring, plumbing, etc.), and the value of the land and building less the amount of any mortgage involved. The salon will usually attempt to rent the residence to which it is connected. Rental income becomes part of the business income.
2. The landlord-salon owner arrangement is also quite common. In this case, the property is owned and maintained by a person who is also the owner and operator of the beauty salon. This landlord-salon owner owns the

land and building, a part of which he or she leases for a beauty salon. He then charges rent to the salon. The value of the salon in this case reflects only the cost of the actual business and not the cost of the structure that houses it.

If the owner of the salon and property lives in a residence, part of which is used for the salon, salon expenses are tax deductible in proportion to the percentage of space occupied by the salon.

Note: Due to our present tax structure, it is wise to consult a good accountant or tax official to find out the best way to set up your accounts in order to take the most advantage of allowable tax deductions.

The home-neighborhood salon is not usually larger than four chairs. The cost of starting such an establishment is quite low, and supplies can be purchased as they are needed. The salon owner-manager is usually the "jack-of-all-trades" . . . receptionist, operator, repairman, bookkeeper, maid, manicurist, public relations person, and supply room clerk. As a result, the percentage of profit shown by a small operation is the highest in our industry, at the cost of a heavier workload and a reduced amount of the owner/manager's free time.

Naming a Beauty Salon

A beauty salon's name should have certain qualities. Some of the most important are:

- It should clearly identify the salon and not be confused with the names of other salons.
- It should be short and memorable.
- It should reflect the image or values of the salon.
- It should not be so trendy that it will become dated when styles change.

Here are examples of salon names and their advantages and disadvantages.

Julie's: The name is a bit informal, and you can't tell from the name that Julie's is a salon. The name has the advantage of being very personal, and that does carry special appeal. If Julie's offers warm, personal service, then the name captures something very important.

Coiffures by Jacques: The name sounds a bit cold, but the place is obviously a salon. If European styling is the specialty here, then the name is appropriate, although it sounds a little corny.

Family Kuts: This sounds like a place to get your hair cut inexpensively. Certainly the name won't attract clients who want to spend a lot of money on their hair or other beauty needs, but they don't expect the stylist to linger over their hair either.

Jackie Fuller's Hair Design Team: Here, the impression is of a very professional, highly motivated, and educated staff. Jackie Fuller's name helps convey a sense of pride and strong personal direction, while the rest of the name shows that the client can expect artistic excellence and a team-oriented approach. The name definitely sounds high-end.

Who Owns the Salon?

Several ownership arrangements have developed in the past several years. They range from individual ownership to a corporation type of arrangement.[1]

Individual Ownership

In this type of salon the owner-manager is directly responsible for the salon's management. Good or bad, the owner makes all the profits or bears the total loss. The owner is responsible for hiring employees.

Usually, the salon runs best when the owner is present. It will run well in the owner's absence only if the staff has been carefully selected and trained to assume responsibility.

Because the staff is loyal to the owner, the individually owned salon usually has little resale value beyond the basic cost of the equipment. Individual owners should not count on making a lot of money by selling at the end of their career.

---

[1] The classes of ownership presented here are simplified for explanation purposes. Before entering into any agreement in ownership of a salon, consult a good attorney in your area. He or she will be able to advise you in legal matters.

Instead, they should set aside money for retirement and emergencies throughout their working career.

In good times an owner has no problem with finances or money. In bad times and slow times of the year, money can be a problem. In single ownership, the salon's entire financial structure is based upon the owner's own personal financial security. While single ownership has many problems, most small salons in our country today are structured this way.

Partnership

This is a marriage of two people in a business venture with a binding contract. When two people are joined together in a business contract, they both are equally responsible for the well-being of the business, thereby giving it more financial security than an individually owned salon. With a partnership, written agreement should set forth definite terms. Some of these are:

1. The amount of money each partner is to invest in setting up the partnership.
2. The amount of time each partner will spend on the business.
3. The exact duties of each partner in relation to the business. (Some of the duties of the partners are given here, but it should be noted that each business has its own kind of problems.) The selection of employees and the assigning of their duties should be the responsibility of one partner. The owners might meet privately and discuss problems of employees, but the employees must know who has the final word concerning their duties. The ordering and control of supplies should be the responsibility of one partner. The advertising program, bookkeeping, salon promotion program, cleaning and maintenance, and decoration and display should all be spelled out in the original partnership agreement.
4. The wages for each partner.
5. How bills are to be paid.
6. How much of an expense account each partner should have.

Each of these items should be written into the contract and changed as needed.

After the contract has been written, rules should be added for the termination of the partnership. Termination might occur upon the death of one of the partners or by ninety days' notice of one of the partners. The cost of purchasing a partner's portion of the business should be stated either in terms of a fixed amount or at the current value. Whether or not a third party can purchase the partner's interest is most important and must be stated.

Some of the good things about a partnership are:

- The joint liability for debts makes the financial structure more sound.
- The salon management is more secure because, when one of the owners is on vacation or is sick, the other owner is present.
- Since there are two or more owners, the actual workload of a single owner is divided.

The one negative feature of a partnership arrangement is that each partner is responsible for anything his or her business partner might do.

The Corporation

In the past, most corporations were large, chain-type operations found in large department stores. In recent years, however, small salon corporations have grown popular and, because of certain tax advantages, may someday completely replace the partnership. In a corporation, several people may invest money in a business and are given stock (shares). In this respect it resembles a partnership. The main difference is in corporate responsibility and termination.

Like a salon under a single owner or partnership, the corporation can buy and sell products, conduct business, pay taxes, make profits, and, in general, function in much the same manner. Other differences are quite striking, however.

A salon that is a corporation can be involved in a lawsuit. However, any resulting damages are levied against the corporation, and individual shareholders are not held responsible. The extent to which a stockholder is responsible for damages is only as great as his stock. Here is an example:

A client wins a malpractice lawsuit against the salon for $15,000.

1. In a single ownership, the owner (or the insurance agent) is responsible for the damages caused on his property. He or she must pay the full amount of the claim even to the extent of selling his or her home, car, and business to do so.
2. In a partnership agreement, each partner is responsible to the extent of his or her ownership in the company. If he or she has two partners (a three-way partnership), each partner would have to pay $5,000.

3. In a corporation, the stockholder is responsible only to the extent of his or her stock. His or her home, automobile, or any other assets cannot be attached. This limited liability is one of the chief advantages of a corporation.

Since stock changes hands as the corporative bylaws permit, owners (stockholders) do not have to be salon personnel. The stockholder invests his money in a salon and receives shares of stock in return. For the use of his money, which he has invested, he receives a dividend at the end of each year (month, week) according to the profits that the salon has made.

Several different types of corporations exist, and each has particular advantages. For example, one person can incorporate his or her business and thereby gain legal protection from personal financial responsibility for the corporation's debts; however, income could conceivably be taxed twice. Talk to a good accountant and a good lawyer before forming any corporation.

The Ownership-Cooperative Corporation

To secure and stabilize help, the single owner forms a corporation in which the stock value reflects the cost of the business plus an added figure (which covers the cost of the owner's work, effort, equipment, and location of the salon). When this figure has been reached, the owner issues the stock, often in the form of employee compensation. More commonly it is made available for employee purchase. The face value can be any figure he wishes. The stock is controlled by the bylaws of the corporation and must be sold back to the corporation upon the termination of the employee. Example:

An owner named John Doe starts a salon with an investment of $15,000 and feels that he has done about $5,000 worth of work in setting up the salon. He thus feels that the salon is worth $20,000. The salon has eight chairs. He then sets up a corporation, called John Doe Beauty Salon, Inc., in which, after one year of employment, an employee can purchase stock. The stock sells at $25 per share, and an employee can purchase as much as he wishes up to $2,000. The stockholder receives a cash dividend at the end of each year on the profits of the salon according to the amount of stock he holds.

Looking at it from John Doe's point of view, John still controls the salon (as long as he controls the majority of the stock). He has employees who will not leave him for another employer because each employee owns part of the business. John can take a vacation knowing that the salon will be left in the hands of another owner. The money John receives from his employees can be used to purchase other stocks and investments or can just earn interest in a bank.

Looking at it from the employee's point of view, he or she is saving money, which can be reclaimed at any time when he or she leaves the corporation. The employee is making more money on the stock (dividends) than could be made keeping his money in a savings account. He or she draws a regular salary as well.

The job is secure because of the corporation contract, which gives a sixty-day notice of termination (even though the contract states that he will give the corporation sixty days' notice of termination). The employee has the pride of ownership in the company without the many problems facing management each day.

Franchise Salons

Franchise salons have expanded significantly over the last fifteen years. Like the food franchise operations (such as McDonald's), these have been very successful because of their marketing and organizational strengths.

Although most of these franchises are locally owned by individuals, some are in fact owned by the franchise company. Regardless, a franchise offers standardization. Management operations and services are all done under strict guidelines to assure a certain level of quality. Decor is standard, as are the products sold and even the design of the salon.

Although such an operation would seem stifling to some people, it has certain advantages:

- Strong consumer advertising.
- Group purchasing power.
- Uniform bookkeeping systems.
- Centralized training.
- Zones guarantee noncompetition from other salons in the same franchise.
- Exclusivity of product line.
- Help with interior design.
- Legal and business assistance programs at a reduced cost.
- Group insurance rates for malpractice and liability.
- Group health insurance for employees.

When you purchase a franchise, you buy into an established name and a system. Be sure you want to be a part of it and that you can generate the income you want. Note also that franchises are for those most interested in the business side of salon ownership.

Employee-Owned Corporation

Employee stock ownership plans offer some unique advantages. In this type of arrangement, the employees own stock in the company, which they purchase when the company is formed or which they earn as part of their compensation over the years. As part owners, they have a strong interest in the success of the entire salon.

Stockholders elect officers. Depending on the bylaws governing the corporation, these officers or others are designated as managers, bookkeeper, etc., and are reimbursed accordingly. Because votes are counted according to how much stock is owned, those with the most stock have the most control. In some cases, the original owner may still hold a controlling interest (51 percent or more) of the stock, while in others the stock is more evenly distributed and decisions are made cooperatively.

A cooperative venture works best when the members know how to work together, of course, and when they realize that compromise is essential. Although not very common, employee ownership is a viable alternative, but only if the personalities involved are compatible. Even with stock being evenly distributed, however, one or two people usually emerge as leaders. Truthfully, even the most agreeable people will have difficulty running a successful salon as a group without the strong guidance of a leader to give the business direction and consistency.

Be Aware, and Beware

The six styles of salon management and ownership presented here do not represent the only types of ownership and management. Creative business people constantly work out new, advantageous hybrids of these and other systems. Before entering into any arrangement, however, you should be aware of four rules that will work to protect your interests:

1. Know what you are purchasing (have it in writing).
2. Know your responsibilities and rights within that agreement.

3. Know how you can terminate the agreement if it becomes necessary.

4. Consult with a good business attorney before entering into any contract. Have him or her read the contract and spell out the advantages and disadvantages for you. Be sure this attorney represents only you and your interests in this arrangement.

CHAPTER ONE SUMMARY

- The four major groups of beauty salons are hotel, department store, shopping center, and home-neighborhood salons.
- A beauty salon's name should clearly identify the salon, be short and memorable, reflect the image or values of the salon, and not be so trendy that it will become dated.
- Ownership arrangements include individual, the partnership, the corporation, the ownership cooperative corporation, franchise salons, and the employee-owned corporation.
- Creative businesspeople develop new, advantageous hybrids of these systems and others.

REVIEW QUESTIONS

1. Where are skin-care services most often found?
2. What is the oldest type of salon existing today?
3. In single ownership, what is the salon's financial structure based on?
4. What sets the franchise apart from other types of salons?
5. Who has the most control in an employee-owned corporation?

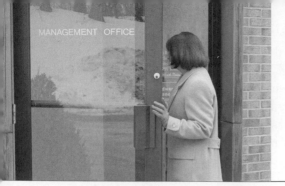

Types of Leases and Rent Agreements

Basic Inclusions

Rent agreements are as simple or as complex as the owner of the property and the renter wish to make them. Complex or simple, they all have certain things in common. They all clearly state the name of the owner and the lessee. All leases contain the day the lease is to start and sometimes actually state the time, such as 12:00 noon. All leases state the day the lease is to expire and sometimes, like the starting clause, the lease may contain an hour of expiration. All leases, regardless of how simple, state the location of the property to be leased, a description thereof, and for what purpose the property is to be used.

Rents are stated as yearly or monthly rates or can be stated as a yearly rate with a percentage clause. The percentage clause means that, after the salon grosses a certain amount of business, the rent will be computed on a percentage of the gross rather than the flat rent fee. Last, all leases contain the signature of both parties and that of a notary public.

Complex Leases

Several other items may appear in more complex leases. These should be carefully read and, if questions arise, discussed with your attorney. Some other items that might be found in a lease are explained in the section that follows:

1. *Returning the property clause:* This generally states that you, as lessee, will return the property to its original condition or better when you vacate the property. In some cases it will state that any improvements that you add must be left intact and in good working order. However, if a beauty salon should place an air conditioner on the property, and provide wiring and ductwork, a lower rent might be requested to offset this expense.

2. *Maintenance clause:* This states who is responsible for the plumbing, heating system, snow removal, window washing, exterior property painting, parking lot cleaning, and major repairs of the property (such as the roof, exterior walls, rain gutters, steps, etc.).

3. *Liability clause for the property:* The salon owner, in some cases, may be responsible not only for the well-being of his clients in the salon but also for the sidewalk and parking area equal to the width of his salon to the street. In the case of a shopping center, it could be several hundred feet.

4. *Sublease clause:* This sometimes becomes quite a problem for a shop wishing to set up a concession and seeking rental income. Since retailing is becoming more of an asset to the beauty business, be sure to find out if you can sell beauty products, clothing, wigs, hats, etc., on this basis.

5. *Major decorating clause:* This could state that in some cases you might need the permission of the owner before you can remodel your salon. If the change is major, you might seek help with the financial cost, which could take the form of rent reduction.

6. *Thirty days' notice clause:* This allows the landlord to show your space to prospective tenants thirty days before you terminate the lease contract. This clause also gives him or her the right to place a For Rent sign in your window thirty days before your lease runs out.

7. *Single business clause:* This states that you will be the only salon in the shopping center or leasing area. In areas where multiple salons are located, the lease may contain a clause stating how close to yours (in feet) the nearest salon may be located. Sometimes the type of salon is noted in the agreement to ensure that a cut-rate salon or beauty school is not located too close to a higher-priced salon.

8. *Deposit clause:* This states that the landlord will hold your deposit money—usually one month's rent—to cover any damage to the property that is not considered normal wear and tear. Protect yourself by noting all damage or missing items before moving in and having the landlord sign a list of these. After you have vacated the premises, the landlord will wait thirty to sixty

days before returning your deposit money to ensure that all debts have been paid.

9. *Property waiver:* Certain property in your salon may not be yours. For example, leased equipment belongs to the company you lease it from. A property waiver will exclude such property from seizure by the landlord and will protect you from having to pay for property you no longer have control over in the event that a dispute with the landlord escalates to seizure of property.

The Tentative Contract

After the space is secured, a tentative contract is signed. A tentative contract is a contract stating that, if the space can pass zoning rules and state board of cosmetology rules and regulations, and you can get a permit for building and redecorating, an electrical permit, a plumbing permit, a sign permit, and any other permits you may need in your locality, on a given date you will sign the lease agreement.

Arranging a Lease

Arranging a lease is a four-step process.

First, select a location convenient to the clientele you wish to serve. Research the location by talking to other business owners in the area. Find out about rent costs per square foot; zoning restrictions; demographics of the people who work, shop, or live in the area; the parking situation; security; problems during bad weather; etc. Get a feel for whether the area is holding steady, improving, or declining, as urban decay could conceivably overtake your salon well before the lease expires.

Second, determine what businesses will help your business. A grocery store or a drugstore, for example, will have a positive influence on your business. A lawyer's office or a mortuary may not. Businesses with a high volume of traffic in which people have a good feeling entering and leaving will have a positive influence. This high-volume traffic will allow you to pay a larger rent, since some of the traffic will spill into your salon.

Third, for the initial meeting with your landlord have ready all information about yourself and the business you wish to operate. This information should include a personal financial profile, your years of experience in the business, educational background, approximate opening date, number of operators you intend to employ, bank references, and lines of credit. The lease may also include the estimated gross sales you project for the business over the next three years.

Fourth, arrange for a tentative contract and first draft of the final lease contract. Both of these should be taken to a lawyer for counsel before signing. Be sure you know how to enter the contract and all the exact do's and don'ts of the lease as well as how to break the lease should the need arise.

CHAPTER TWO SUMMARY

- All leases state certain things: the owner's and lessee's names, the day and sometimes the time the lease begins, the day and sometimes the time the lease expires, and the location and description of the property and for what purpose the property will be used.
- Additional items may appear in more complex leases and these should be carefully read.
- Arranging a lease is a four-step process: selecting a location, determining what businesses will help your business, showing the landlord all pertinent information about yourself, and arranging for a tentative contract and first draft of the final lease.

REVIEW QUESTIONS

1. Who must sign a lease in addition to the two parties involved?
2. What does a deposit clause state?
3. What businesses might help your business?
4. Before you sign the final lease, who should look at it?

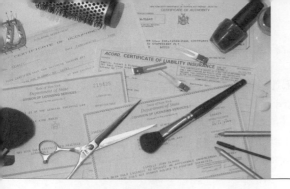

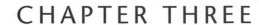

Permits, Public Utilities, and Insurance

Permits

Because of their importance, we shall discuss necessary permits and where to obtain them.

1. *Permission from the state board of cosmetology:* This board is usually found at the state capitol or an annex thereof. Permission can be obtained by letter or in person, and upon request they will give you a set of salon and operator rules and regulations. In some states you receive a salon license without delay. More likely, the state board will request a salon plan, which shows the arrangement of the working area, the general arrangement of the supply area, toilet space, doors (interior and exterior), windows or a ventilation system, and other such information as is required by that state.

2. *Plumbing permit:* This can be obtained by a plumbing contractor and added to his bill, or you can secure it for him. The permit is usually obtained at the city hall in the office of the zoning and building inspector.

3. *Electrical permit:* This can be obtained at the city hall in the office of the zoning and building inspector by you or your electrical contractor.

4. *Sign permit:* This can be obtained by you or a sign contractor at the office of

the zoning and building inspector at the city hall. Some cities are very restrictive about what size and type of signs may be displayed, especially in areas designated as historic.

5. *Building permit:* Plans showing the construction of walls and the materials to be used will be necessary. You can obtain this for yourself or have your building contractor get it. It, like the other permits, can be obtained from your city's zoning and building inspector. If the building site contains asbestos, it will have to be removed at considerable expense. If removal is necessary, be sure that the landlord will pay for this procedure. Also, be sure to have the building inspected for electrical wiring problems, water damage, and structural damage caused by termites or other vermin.

6. *Zoning permit:* Be sure to check on the zoning rules in the area where you intend to locate the salon. This is important because, if the zoning is not correct for that type of business, you may have to make an appeal to have the zoning laws changed or obtain a variance. If you have to change the zoning laws, you will have to spend much time, effort, and, in some cases, money. Be sure your landlord helps to defray this cost because it will affect his whole property. This can be done in the office of the zoning and building inspector in your city.

7. *Sales tax license:* This can be obtained from the finance department in the city sales tax division. Without this license you cannot sell any retail item in your salon. A record of sales for retail must be made and kept for this department.

8. *State sales tax:* All businesses must have a sales tax number. This can be applied for from the revenue department in your state. A sales tax number is usually applied for by a bookkeeper or an accountant. Accounts for taxes on employee earnings can be set up at this time as well.

9. *Use tax:* Certain cities have a use tax on items purchased in another city and used by you to make a profit. An example is a hair dryer purchased in Denver, Colorado, to be used in Boulder, Colorado. The city of Boulder can collect a tax on that dryer in the form of a use tax. Be sure to check on use tax in your area. The information can be obtained at the city office of finance.

10. *Vending machines:* If you are going to have a candy machine, soda machine, or any other type of vending machine, you may need an additional license. Check with your local department of revenue and finance to learn if one is needed.

Securing Public Utilities

Securing public utilities varies from town to town and from state to state. For the most part, the plumbing, electrical, and building contractors will take care of the major requirements. They are the experts about size of wire, pipe, and units that will be required. They will connect you to public utilities, and all you have to do is to secure and start service.

In some places, the gas and electric companies are combined, and one stop will take care of both. You will want to know how much your service will cost per month. An estimate will sometimes be used. If you do not already have credit with these companies, a deposit may be required. This deposit can be as much as three months' service. After a year of continuous service, the company will usually refund the deposit. In some cases, but not all, your deposit will earn interest. Most utilities will want your name, address, the name and nature of the business, and three credit references.

For new accounts, the telephone company will require a deposit that will be held for six months to a year. This deposit is not unusual, but, again, the amount of money required and the length of time the telephone company will hold it depends upon the company and its location.

There is a standard charge for phone installation, and this charge includes your name in both the white and Yellow pages of the local phone directories. Each additional phone installation is an added charge, but you can purchase your own phone. If you would like to advertise in the Yellow pages, this can be arranged for an additional charge plus a regular monthly fee for the ad.

You can determine the many other services that your phone company offers by placing a call to the business accounts office.

Arrangements with the water company are usually taken care of by the land-lord; however, it is most important that you, as a salon owner, know who pays the bill. If you are responsible for paying the water bill, it is advisable to stop by the water office and apply for service about two weeks in advance of opening. They, like the other utility companies, may require a deposit. The forms used are quite simple and should not take more than a few minutes to fill out.

The trash removal service is usually arranged by the salon unless stated differently in the lease agreement. This company is contacted by telephone as soon as you move into the salon. All that is normally needed is a statement that you wish service. They will ask your name and address, the name of the business and its address, and when service should start. Some trash services furnish their own containers. If you furnish your own trash container, be sure that it meets with local and state regulations of the state board of cosmetology, the fire department, and the department of sanitation.

Environmental regulations have become very strict in many areas. Check with local authorities to be sure that your salon will meet the local codes, especially regarding what is poured down the drain. Also, mandated recycling programs call for you to separate certain items from your trash and place these in different containers for collection.

The last thing you should do before moving into your salon is to contact your local fire and police departments. The two departments will want to know who owns the salon, where they can be reached, and when the salon is open for business. After you have your staff set up, it would be wise to give an additional name to the fire and police departments, just in case you cannot be reached during an emergency.

Insurance

A contract of insurance is an agreement whereby an insurance company, for a consideration called a premium, agrees to compensate the insured for loss or damage to the insured's property or agrees to protect the insured against legal liability. There are two general classifications of insurance: indemnity insurance and liability insurance. *Indemnity insurance* provides for payment by the insurance company to the insured for any losses suffered as a result of damage to the insured's property or person. *Liability insurance* provides protection for the insured for losses resulting from legal liability. If a person is hurt on the insured's premises and sues for damages, the insured has a legal liability.

Types of Insurance

Arrange meetings with several independent insurance agents. These specialists write contracts for many companies, so they can select from many policies to formulate insurance for your specific needs. Comparison shop among the various proposals, since by doing so you should be able to save 10 to 15 percent of your total insurance budget.

During these meetings, have each agent provide you with insurance proposals as well as safety check sheets regarding inspection of equipment, physical structures, and protection of the public. Check insurance proposals for cancellation clauses and increased rates due to claims. Check to see if cancellation is automatic after a number of claims have been made during a policy year. Find out if claims are honored for out-of-court as well as in-court settlements. Check the amount you will receive during the time these settlement cases or court deliberations keep you away from the salon. Also ask who would pay the costs of witnesses and other related expenses.

Use the various types of insurance coverage discussed in this section as a guide to determine your specific policy needs.

Fire. This type of insurance covers an individual for losses resulting from damage to property as a result of a fire. Fire insurance is a basic form of coverage that most businessmen carry.

80 Percent Coinsurance Clause: In order that the insured carries sufficient coverage to protect himself or herself from a partial loss, a coinsurance clause (usually 80 percent) has become a standard feature of most fire insurance policies. This clause makes it mandatory that the insured carries at least 80 percent of the value of the property in insurance. The failure to carry this amount of insurance automatically makes the insured a coinsurer for any partial losses.

Liability. This covers a person who has an accident on your property or the space for which you are responsible. Accidents happen when people slip on an icy sidewalk or a wet floor. The cost of this type of insurance is reasonable considering the broad span of coverage offered.

Malpractice. This protects the salon and operators against suits resulting from injury due to neglect or misuse of a product while a service is being rendered. The cost of this insurance varies as you increase the number of employees in the salon and the services that the salon performs.

Equipment and Supply. This covers damage, other than normal wear and tear, to everything in the salon.

Example:

The salon is broken into, and vandalism occurs, resulting in mirrors being broken, chairs ripped, and supplies dumped. The resulting loss would be covered. The cost of such insurance varies with location, value of equipment at time of policy renewal, and various other clauses the owner wishes to insert.

Theft, Burglary, and Robbery. These are all types of insurance that indemnify the insured for losses resulting from a criminal act.

Theft insurance: Losses resulting from the disappearance of valuables or money.

Burglary insurance: Losses resulting as a result of forced, illegal entry into the premises when they are closed.

Robbery insurance: Losses resulting from the use of force or the threat of force.

Compensation. Most states have enacted legislation to provide for coverage of employees who are injured as a result of accidents in the course of employment. In most states this coverage is mandatory, and anyone who employs people is legally obligated to carry it.

Business Interruption. This form of insurance can be written as a separate policy or added to some other form of insurance, such as fire or equipment and supply insurance. It is written to cover anticipated losses due to the interruption of business as a result of fire or some other catastrophe. Employees' loss of income can also be covered so employees do not desert the employer while business is interrupted.

Health. This is sometimes offered as a benefit to individuals in the salon under a group plan. The salon may or may not pay a part of the premium. The AIDS health crisis has caused some insurance companies to stop issuing health insurance policies to salons because of the stereotype that male homosexuals are disproportionately represented in the salon profession. If you are denied insurance, check with your state insurance agency to see what your legal recourses are.

FICA (Social Security). All salons are required to withhold FICA taxes from an employee's wages. For information on FICA rules and regulations, contact the Internal Revenue Service. Your accountant can do this for you and fill out the necessary forms.

Loss of Income (Disability). This insurance covers the wages of an operator in case of accident and/or illness. Usually the salon does not cover employees in this area but leaves this coverage to the individual employee to handle privately.

CHAPTER THREE SUMMARY

- A number of permits must be obtained before a salon can be opened.
- Plumbing, electrical, and building contractors can connect you to public utilities; you will need to arrange for service to start.
- Prospective salon owners should find out about both indemnity and liability insurance from several independent insurance agents.

REVIEW QUESTIONS

1. What must be done if a building site contains asbestos?
2. What is a use tax?
3. What protection does liability insurance provide?
4. Why should you have equipment and supply insurance?
5. Who must withhold FICA taxes?

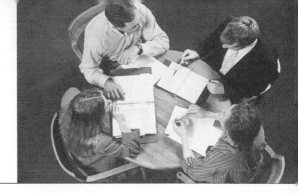

CHAPTER FOUR

Financing the New Salon

Sources of Money

Unfortunately, most people do not have a rich uncle. So before opening a beauty salon, the owner must face the problem of financing.

Equity vs. Financed Capital

One of the first financial decisions you must make is how much of your salon will be equity, how much will be financed, and whether to borrow funds. Changes in the tax laws have practically eliminated the advantages of leasing equipment over borrowing capital. Look closely at all costs, add up total costs, and then see whether leasing or a loan is more affordable.

Your total cash situation will make a difference. If you are cash poor or will be needing cash reserves in the foreseeable future, leasing may be the better option because you will not have to put any money down. If you have plenty of cash, you can reduce the amount you pay each month by making a large down payment—and your total costs will be less.

Consult with your accountant before making any final decision.

Banks

If you wish to obtain a bank loan, you may have some difficulty. The bank must secure a loan with something. A salon that hasn't opened, doesn't have working operators or a reputation; at this point, the salon is nothing but a dream on paper and is not financially secure. When considering a loan to a person for a salon, a bank will take a careful look at the owner's personal finances. It will, no doubt, want to know what property you own, what you owe to creditors, the names of firms with whom you have credit, your past five years' income tax statements, your experience in the field, who you are going to hire, and how much money you will need. In most cases, the bank would rather secure the loan with a house, car, stocks, bonds, or furniture than on a beauty salon and equipment. This is because salon furniture and equipment have few outlets for resale. In the case of default of payments, the bank gets the salon furniture and equipment but has a difficult time finding a customer for it.

Several loan agencies across the country will finance salons. Their interest rates are usually so high that it is best to forget this outlet for finance.

Local distributors and major manufacturers will lease you equipment and supplies. Their interest rates may be less than those of a bank or loan agency. Securing a loan from a supply dealer is far less difficult because, if the salon should go bankrupt, it is in a better position to repossess and dispose of the equipment.

Some distributors have engineers who will design your salon for you. They will draw up a set of plans, showing location of equipment, electrical outlets, plumbing, and heating systems. This is done without charge in most cases if you purchase your equipment from them. If you want only the plans, the supply house will charge a fee for this service. Before starting a salon in any area, consult your leading distributor. It will be most helpful in getting you established.

Used equipment sells for 25 to 60 percent of its original value. If it suits your needs and your style, you can save a substantial sum if you buy used equipment. Be sure that this equipment is in good working order and that you have enough of each item to complete your needs. Beware of equipment that needs repair; your repair costs and the inconvenience involved may cancel out any savings.

Beauty supply distributors are good sources of used equipment. They can guarantee the integrity and can loan you equipment if yours fails. If you purchase equipment directly from a salon or other source, be very careful. Here are some of the problems you may encounter:

1. The equipment was not owned by the salon, but was only leased, or was subject to a lien by the bank.
2. The purchase doesn't include all the fixtures. For example, you purchase a shampoo sink and learn that the plumbing doesn't go with it.
3. Is there a sales or use tax on the purchase? If you take it across a state line, do you need a permit or do you have to pay another tax?

Equipment

You will most likely be selecting your equipment according to the style and color you like. But there are a few practical decisions you must make. First, do you want an almost private salon with booths or an "open air" salon where everyone works out in the open? Second, do you want wet styling stations (with shampoo bowl and styling station together) or a dry station with a wet section in the salon (shampoo bowls in one area)? There are positive and negative features with each arrangement.

Third, do you want to serve both men and women (unisex)? The style of equipment, arrangement, and aesthetic decor will vary with this decision. Fourth, do you wish to operate a full-service salon with nail care, skin care, and perhaps a boutique with clothing items? Planning ahead is easier than trying to expand later. These are major decisions that will determine the entire atmosphere of the salon or styling center.

CHAPTER FOUR SUMMARY

- One of the first financial decisions you must make is how much of the salon will be equity, how much will be financed, and whether to borrow money.
- A bank, when asked to finance a new business, will look carefully at the owner's personal finances.
- Selection of equipment will depend on several decisions: whether the salon will be private or "open air," whether there will be wet or dry styling stations, whether the salon will serve both men and women, and whether the salon will be full-service.

REVIEW QUESTIONS

1. When is leasing definitely a better option?
2. In most cases, what do banks like to use to secure loans?
3. For what percentage of original value does used equipment sell?
4. What do wet styling stations combine?

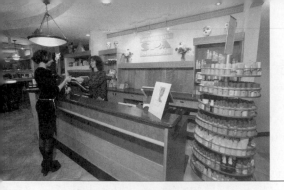

Decorating and Arranging the Reception Area

First impressions are lasting impressions. No better saying could open this chapter. What makes a good impression? The reception room is the first place a person will see when entering the salon and the last place the client will remember when leaving. It should have a quality of saying, "Hello, you are welcome here," and "Relax and enjoy yourself." When the client leaves the salon, the room should say, "Please come back, thank you, and return soon."

Your front window, properly arranged, is one of the salon's best assets. Designed effectively, displays in a shop window will increase walk-in business by as much as 50 percent. Display advertising is not new; department stores, grocery stores, and many other successful businesses spend thousands of dollars on this form of advertising. On a street heavily traveled with foot traffic, window displays are necessary to attract customers.

Windows

Here are several rules to follow when decorating your windows:

1. *Windows should be cleaned at least once a week.* Hair spray on the inside of windows quickly clouds the glass and make it dull. Weekly cleaning will keep the glass shining, clear, and easy to maintain.

2. *Window drapes should be cleaned regularly* and should add warmth and privacy to a salon. Set up a drapery cleaning schedule and have the drapes cleaned at least once every six months.

3. *Window displays should stress one theme,* and preferably one item. It is better to have one item displayed well than a hundred items competing with each other.

4. *A hairstyle display card should be included.* It should be easy to read and contain only a few words: "Style by Mr. Edward," "Style of the Month," "Season's Greetings," "Sail into Spring with a New Wave," "Swing into Spring with a New Hairstyle," "Color Makes the Difference."

5. *Displays should be changed regularly.* In this business it is suggested that displays change every month to two months.

6. *Promote your image in the window* to entice walk-ins. Also, remember the powerful lure of the words *Free, Complimentary, Gift,* etc. Your window is your most valuable tool for luring walk-in clients who may then become regular visitors.

Door

Your main door is almost as important as your window. In most cases, the door should contain the name of the salon, leaving the window for display. In some cases, all doors in the area are the same. Regardless of this, yours can be decorated to make it different.

All doors should have the following characteristics:

1. They should look appealing.
2. They should be clean and well kept.
3. They should be easy to open by the client.
4. They should be wide enough for a wheelchair to pass through without undue stress.
5. If possible, they should swing in and out. Some cities have a fire law that states that all business establishments must have doors that swing out. Check your local fire code.
6. If they are glass, they should be made of shatterproof glass, with a design on the doors to help prevent people from walking into them.

Where Do I Put My Coat?

The Coat Rack

Coat trees are impractical and ugly when overburdened, making a coat rack preferable. A good coat rack with sturdy plastic or wooden hangers is a necessity. Be sure that the rack is out of the way but within sight of the receptionist (for security). The best design is one that includes a rack above for hats and a rack on the sides for umbrellas.

The Coat Closet

This is a really good idea with two problems: first, they cost money to build and, second, any time you enclose damp clothes you are bound to create odors that will affect everyone's clothing in that area.

   The best solution seems to be a compromise between a closet and a coat rack. This can be built on a stationary wall, and consists of two supports and a pole. A shelf above is a must for hats and packages carried by clients. Because this area is open at the top, no musty odors will accumulate. The area should be close to the receptionist's desk, making it easy for him or her to hang up clients' coats when they arrive. A light in that area is a must. Clothes hangers should be made of wood or sturdy plastic. These will support the weight of a winter coat as well as a sweater. Metal hangers often leave creases in heavy clothing and tend to bend and sag. Wooden hangers can be purchased at a reasonable cost and should be replaced when needed

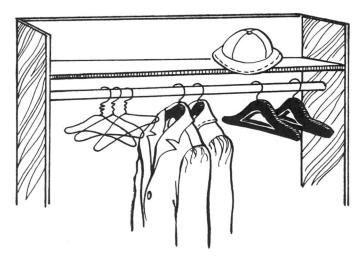

Magazines, Books, and Newspapers

Before selecting magazines for your salon, be sure to study your clients. If you mainly serve the housewife, be sure your magazines reflect this. If you cater to young people, you may have magazines such as *Seventeen*, *Vogue*, and *Glamour*. A good rule to use in selecting magazines is "select the same percentage of a type of magazine as the percentage of customers." This means that, if 10 percent of your customers are teenagers, 10 percent of your magazines will be for them.

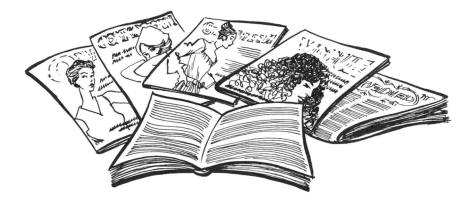

In selecting the number of magazines for your salon, a good rule is "three magazines for each operator." A shop of six operators would have eighteen magazines. These magazines can be purchased by subscription at a lower price than if they were obtained at a newsstand.

Magazines should be changed at least once a month. No magazine should remain in the beauty salon beyond a month after its publication date. Plastic covers for your magazines are available and will keep your magazines looking good for a long time. These covers come in a number of colors and should be changed as the seasons are changed. If plastic covers are used, the cover can be used to advertise certain special services.

A suggested cross section of magazines for a six-chair beauty salon includes:

3 movie magazines
2 fashion magazines
3 general information magazines
2 men's magazines
2 women's magazines
2 news magazines

2 house magazines
1 cooking magazine
2 travel magazines

For salons with a high number of male clients:

1 *Gentlemen's Quarterly*
1 *Popular Mechanics*
2 sports magazines
1 *Esquire*

The local newspaper should be in all salons. A few paperback books on cooking, meal planning, hobbies, or arts and crafts are also good to have around.

Magazines should be placed on a table or a magazine rack. They should never be left on chairs or the floor. A good receptionist will replace these after the client has left the area.

Children's Area

In neighborhood salons, mothers will often bring their children with them. To avoid accidents involving children in the styling area, possibly leading to a lawsuit, a children's area in the waiting area is sometimes provided. A sign placed at the entrance of the styling area, **"For Safety's Sake Children Must Remain Seated in the Waiting Area or Reception Area,"** usually keeps them out of the work area. The children's area should be on one side of the waiting room and oriented so the children are out of the way of the rest of the clients of the salon.

A children's area should have the following:

1. A low table, which can be found in the toy department of any leading department store. Be sure this table is well built and sturdy.
2. Four chairs for the table. These should be painted and easy to clean and care for.
3. Several paper doll books, precut.
4. Several plastic cars and trucks. These should be large enough for the children to play with but small enough to be used on their table.
5. Several story books for different age groups.
6. A selection of inexpensive, quiet toys for children of various ages.

7. Avoid crayons and coloring books, as crayons tend to break and children have a habit of coloring the walls.

The items in the children's area should be washable and easy to clean. All items should be easily replaced at little cost.

The receptionist should be made responsible for the actions of the children. She or he should have the right to correct children and maintain order. If the client objects to this arrangement, then the client should be asked to leave his or her children at home. In some larger salons the sign "Children Are Welcome As Customers Only" makes it clear that the salon is a place of relaxation and beauty only.

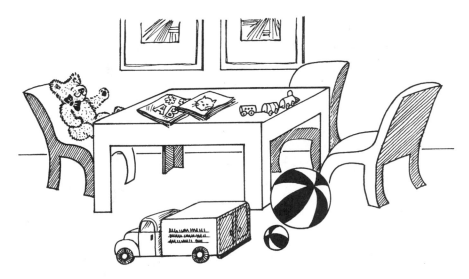

Reception Room Walls

Reception room walls can be of almost any type. They can be painted, paneled, bricked, papered, or almost any other composition you desire.

The color of your walls and draperies affects a salon's waiting room. A good interior designer can help in this regard. A few simple rules follow:

- To make a room appear larger, paint it white or a light color.
- To make a long room look shorter and more square, paint one or two of the smaller walls a darker color. An accent color on one of the walls, with the other wall being white, will also make that wall appear closer.

- If a room has a low ceiling, paint or decorate the walls with vertical stripes. This will make the walls or ceiling appear higher.
- If you wish to cut down the height of a room, decorate it with horizontal lines and pictures.

Draperies can add a whole new dimension to your salon. Consult a good drapery designer to find out how to drape your window. Avoid velvet and velvetlike drapes. They will collect hair spray and dust too rapidly. A light drape will add color and life to the salon. A dark drape will do the opposite and will sometimes make your employees feel listless.

Should you decide to paint your salon, paint the walls with a high-grade, washable paint. This will enable you to clean more easily when needed. For the top part of the wall, you can use a water-based paint and save money.

White paint and white ceilings will make your salon appear clean and light. In most cases, the lighter the salon, the better it is for the morale of the operators and customers.

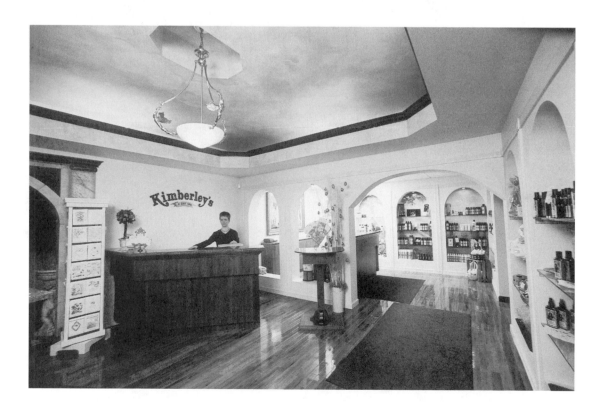

If you use wallpaper, make it blend as the basic color of the salon. A small, muted pattern is much better than a bold one, since it will not dominate the room in which it is placed. A picture placed on a boldly papered wall will lose its effect and so will any advertising display you place on that type of wall. A good rule is to "make it light, bright, but quiet."

Wood panels are very popular. They are easy to install and easy to maintain, and they look good. If wooden walls are used, be sure that they complement the woods or furniture you have in the salon. Some salons can use dark panels, but light wood is easier to keep clean and neat. Light wood will not show scratches and wear as much as dark wood.

If you intend to hang anything on a wood-paneled wall, be sure to have a support for it behind the panel. Otherwise, the whole panel might come away from the wall. The only really bad thing about wood paneling is that it cannot be repaired, only replaced. If your salon has wood paneling, be sure where you drive a nail because the hole will always be there.

Ceramic tile walls have been used in a few salons, usually in the wet section of the salon. While these walls do not require constant repair and can be kept clean with very little effort, they are not often used because they are quite expensive.

Brick walls and brick room dividers are used in a good number of beauty salons. In some cases they are painted, and in other cases they are left exposed and natural. They do not need any special maintenance other than the cost of painting them or an occasional dusting with a vacuum sweeper.

Mirrors are a good idea for one wall of your salon. They will make the salon appear larger and will make any displays appear larger and more pronounced. Mirrors usually come with a stick-on back so they can be installed quickly and with very little effort. A good wiping with soap and water will keep the mirror wall looking good. The maintenance on this type of wall is minor.

Hairstyle pictures or posters should be hung in a reception room. At least two large pictures (3′ × 4′) should be displayed. These pictures and your display wall or cabinet should dominate the entire room. A note on a card or ribbon reading "Hair styled by Mr. Joseph" or "Hairstyle by Miss Jayne" will increase the demand for that person's work. The *Style of the Month* is a good theme to display in the salon. Pictures should be dusted regularly and changed monthly and should definitely have a message.

Photos of styles done in the salon are an effective advertisement for your stylists, but they are expensive (especially since they should be changed every two months) and require specialized photographic skills to look truly professional. For this reason, posters are the better choice for most salons.

A heavy gold or black frame will accent any picture. A picture without a frame will never attract your patrons. Pictures with messages always have a way of selling themselves to the public. A small light, placed on the picture at night, will serve as a night light and also advertise the salon to those who walk by and look in.

Caution: In large cities and shopping centers, the local fire department may have fire codes affecting such things as wallpaper and salon decorations. For example, Christmas trees may have to be fireproof. Always check the fire codes before you invest money and effort on expensive wall coverings and decorations.

Displays

Whether your displays and retail racks hang on the wall or are freestanding, be sure they are accessible to the clients. Customers should be able to pick up, touch, read, and even smell products. If the display is placed behind the receptionist, you will lose more money in sales than you will lose to shrinkage when the racks are accessible.

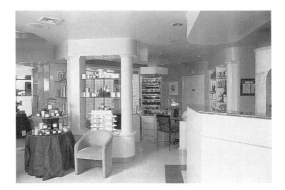

The displays should be located close to the receptionist so she or he can offer advice and answer questions. A display of inexpensively priced, eye-catching items next to the cash register will stimulate impulse buying. Of course, jewelry and small items should be kept close to the reception area, as these are prone to pilferage. If you carry expensive boutique items, these should be in a locked display case but located close to the receptionist so she can show them and maintain control without having to leave her desk.

It should be easy and fast to clean. The backdrop of the display should be easy to change and should be kept current with accent colors.

Shelves in the display section of this wall should be at least six inches deep, but no deeper than eight inches. Good displays are limited to one or two major ideas. It is better to display one item well than several items poorly. Displays on a display wall should be changed about every four to eight weeks.

Displays need to be immaculately kept, fully stocked, attractively arranged, and very well lit. Ask your distributor for advice on setting up displays that sell products. Use your creativity and that of all your employees to make your displays as enticing and varied as possible. Observe how upscale department stores display similar items and borrow their ideas. Use seasonal themes. Above all, avoid having it look crowded or cluttered.

Lighting

Without planning and forethought, lighting in a reception room can be a problem. Five common types of lighting can be successfully adapted for salon use. The type selected will depend upon salon design.

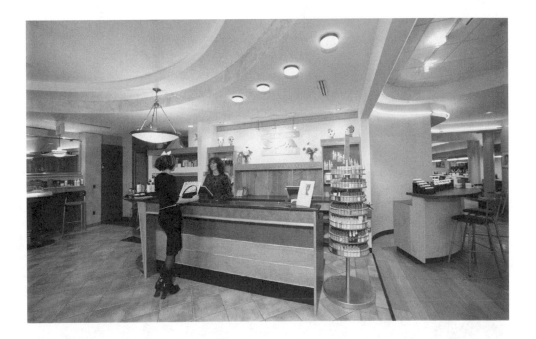

Ceiling lights are very popular. A recessed ceiling light is flush with the ceiling and will not compete with light falling on your displays; however, it will not give off much light. You will find that, if you intend to light your reception room with recessed lights, you will need quite a few of them.

Spotlight or track lighting, either recessed or suspended, can be directed on pictures and displays. This light will definitely increase sales as well as add more light to the reception area. One bad thing about recessed lights and spotlights is that they cannot be moved. As a result you must plan where they should go before they are installed.

Fluorescent tube lights produce the most light and are cheapest to operate. They do not direct your attention to any part of the reception area and are not really noticed by clients. They do very little for the decor of the room. When mirrors are present in the reception area, be sure that tubes selected give off warm tones that are flattering to the complexion. Special fluorescent lighting is now available to correct the blue or green effect of the standard tube. The

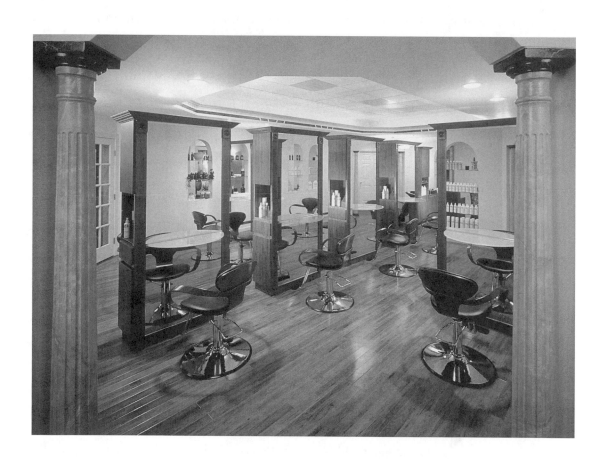

new tubes give almost perfect reproduction of sunlight and can be ordered from any good lighting supplier. Adding a pink and a baby blue light tube along with the standard lighting will have a similar effect.

Chandeliers are used for their beauty and to give light. They add a certain dignity and mood to a salon that enhance the overall decor. Chandeliers should be cleaned and dusted weekly to keep them looking attractive. They should not be so large that they steal attention from displays. In selecting a chandelier, be sure that it is easy to clean. If it is a crystal chandelier, be sure that the prisms can be replaced if they are broken during cleaning. Remember, the simpler the design, the easier it will be to clean.

Wall lighting consists of two types: indirect lighting and wall sconces. Indirect lighting is usually a tube light covered by a box or panel, which directs the light toward the wall or ceiling. This type of fixture gives a soft lighting effect, but a good deal of light is lost because of the covering. If a concealed type of indirect lighting is used, and you anticipate having clients read, be sure that it contains a reflector to aid in directing as much light as possible into the room. Sconces are usually in the form of candles on either side of a picture or a display. Wall lights normally do not give off much light and are used mostly as a decoration or to create special effects.

Table or floor lamps are not commonly used. First, they must be put on a table; second, they might be knocked over by children. If the lamp is large enough to give off enough light to make it an asset, it usually is so large that a large table will be necessary in order for it to look right. When you are renting floor space by the square foot, it is unwise to take up too much space with tables (three tables, which would hold lamps large enough to light a waiting room, would consume as much space as a styling station and a hair dryer). If a table lamp is used, be sure it can be wiped clean either by a damp cloth or with a dust cloth. It should be possible to clean the shade of such a lamp with a damp cloth as hair spray will build up on it.

The Reception Desk

This desk is the nerve center of the salon and controls all its activities. A poorly organized desk will cost many hours of wasted time on the part of your receptionists and operators. As such, it is the most important piece of furniture in the reception room.

The receptionist's desk should be about four feet wide (larger desks are needed in larger salons). A four-foot desk is capable of servicing two to fourteen operators with no problem.

A check-writing stand at the front of the desk should be at least six inches wide. This will enable clients to write a check or place a purse while they pay their bill.

The desk table should be four feet wide and two feet deep. A space for the receptionist's chair should be found at the left and shelves and drawers to the right. The top drawer should be one-and-a-half feet wide and should be as deep as the desk. It should be divided into two sections. The first section is used as a cash drawer, and the second is used as a safe with a key. This drawer should be three inches deep, and the outside of the drawer should also have a lock and key.

Computer systems are appearing in many more salons. Since these may automate functions such as keeping the appointment book, the desk should be arranged accordingly. Also, salon business computers typically include a cash drawer, which may or may not be a part of a separate desk.

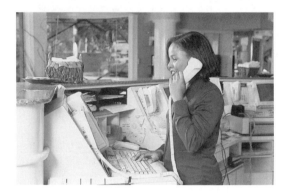

Below the cash drawer should be a file drawer. This should be large enough to hold a file folder. The same width as your cash drawer (a foot-and-a-half) is recommended.

Desk Accessories. On the desk table you should have:

1. *A telephone.* This is usually placed on the left side of the desk so the receptionist can hold it with her left hand and write with her right. A telephone mounted on the side of the desk is better. This will keep it out of the way and will discourage clients from using the phone. (Most clients will not ask a receptionist to dial a number.) An added convenience for the busy receptionist is a headset-type telephone that will allow free use of both hands

while answering the phone. Though not inexpensive, such a phone accessory will prevent stiff neck muscles and dropped phones that can occur otherwise and will allow the receptionist to work more quickly.

2. *An appointment book* large enough for your business and easy to flip from day to day.

3. *A container with several pens and pencils.* A larger eraser is also a good idea. Pencils and pens have a habit of walking away with your customers. Those having your beauty salon name on them are good advertising items.

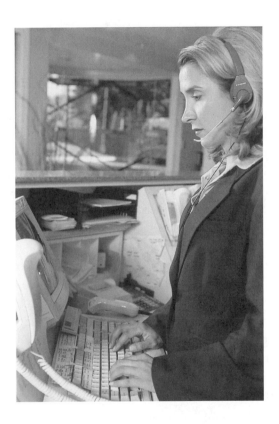

4. *An adding machine*, to check sales tickets and merchandise sales, should be placed on the far right of the desk. If you use a cash register in your salon, it should be placed at the far right of the desk, and the adding machine should be put in the shelf-drawer at the bottom of the desk.

5. *A box of appointment cards.* An appointment card should be given to each client as he or she leaves the salon.

6. *A scratch pad* for notes and messages should be available at all times.

7. A *price list* should be placed on the top of the desk table and be secured to the surface with tape. This is done so that the receptionist will always know where to look when quoting prices.

8. A *phone number and address file* for numbers frequently called should be placed near the telephone and updated every four months.

9. *Operator's ticket holder or file* should be placed at the very rear of the desk and out of the way of conducting business. A letter holder for incoming mail should also be placed next to the ticket holder, and mail should be removed daily.

10. *Computer.* The computer system normally consists of four items: the monitor, the computer keyboard, the computer hardware unit, and the printer. The monitor is normally placed to the left or above the keyboard. It may take the place of the appointment book and adding machine. The computer hardware unit can be placed below the reception desk and the printer next to the filing cabinet. Remember to provide adequate electrical support to the computer components with a special dedicated electrical outlet and electrical breaker. This electrical outlet and breaker will prevent interruptions due to overloaded lines used in the styling area. An additional telephone line is needed for the computer so that the salon's service lines are not overloaded. For more information on computer operation, see Management Information Systems (MIS).

Nothing else should ever be put on the top of this desk; to do so will make it messy.

Below the desk table, the receptionist should have a wastebasket that is large enough to be useful but small enough not to interfere with her feet when she is seated at the desk. A pencil sharpener can be attached to the side of the desk. One should also be placed in the supply room (thereby eliminating any congestion at the desk caused by people sharpening pencils).

The file cabinet drawer should contain the following items, neatly filed:

1. job application forms
2. interview sheets
3. operator evaluation sheets
4. operator's check sheets
5. job application forms, which have been filled out but not used
6. soft drink and vending machine receipt forms
7. operator daily report sheets

8. salon daily report sheets
9. newspaper ads on the salon
10. public relations files
11. supply company's files
12. inventory report forms
13. supply order forms

Note: Even if reports and forms are part of the computer system's operations, a hard copy (paper) should be on file so that management can study reports and discuss needed information with others without having to interfere with the salon's daily activities on the computer. This also eliminates the need for a receptionist to print out reports while trying to serve clients.

The bottom shelf-drawer should hold the extras:

1. extra operator's cash receipt book
2. extra appointment cards
3. extra pencils
4. extra scrap paper
5. extra tint and permanent wave cards
6. erasers
7. a telephone book

Management Information Systems (MIS)

Computer companies would lead a salon owner to believe that no business in the twenty-first century can exist without the aid of a computer. The truth is that the barber/cosmetology industry existed for thousands of years before computers were invented and will continue to thrive with or without these marvelous machines.

Computer specialists are quick to point out that the computer can perform many business functions at speeds that boggle the minds of most salon employees. Often computers are sold to salons under the assumption that the time spent on management functions and record keeping will be reduced. This is not true. A salon of four to six operators fully utilizing a computer system to handle all business transactions would require a person to spend two to three hours a day inputting information. Most salon personnel (hairdressers, manicurists, cosmetologists, and barbers) are not computer experts, nor are they so inclined. Most salon personnel are highly trained and skilled technical experts in the areas of hair, skin, nails, and grooming techniques with great social skills and with little or no desire to be confined to a desk or machine. The mismatch of computers and salon personnel has left most salons using only one or two computer programs, usually for appointments and customer records.

Computer Functions

Besides appointment management and customer records the following are just a few computer capabilities:

- inventory
- personnel records
- bookkeeping
- payroll records
- tax records and payments
- check writing
- making deposits
- bill paying
- ordering of supplies
- manufacturer's information on products
- advertising and promotion
- salon safety records
- development of profit and loss statements

Review the forms mentioned throughout this text. Make a list of all information and functions that you want the computer to perform. Then consult a computer expert for help. All computers and computer software will have trouble at one time or another. Keep the same computer expert for all your computer needs. Like the physician whom you have used for years and who knows your health problems, a computer expert who helped design and put your system into functioning order can be an important ally.

Computer experts often try to make programs easy for themselves. Remember the adage, "He who has the gold makes the rules." You need to tell the computer expert exactly what you want and how you want the computer to do it. It is his or her job to design software to be user friendly to your particular salon.

All the information on a salon's computer should not be available to all salon employees.

Example:

Robert should not be able to access Ann's personnel records, salary information, or performance evaluations. Some information should be available to only a few employees or the owner, while other information (e.g., appointment scheduling) should be available to all salon personnel. Computer specialists can "lock out" certain information so only those persons with a "need to know" will be able to access certain information.

Examples of Computer Usage

Appointments and Scheduling. These programs can be purchased and usually show the days of the week with times of appointments in half-hour blocks, starting at 9:00 A.M. and running to 6:00 P.M. Since some salons open at 6:00 A.M. to get working clients to the office by 8:00 A.M. and often close at 10:00 P.M., the over-the-counter package may not be an answer. A computer programmer can tailor this program for your salon, so the appointment calendar will start each day at 6:00 A.M. and run through 10:00 P.M. Services can also be programmed so that when a patron schedules a permanent wave that requires two hours to complete, adequate time will automatically be blocked out. Special appointment time at the end of the day will allow an operator to add additional appointments that the computer may not be programmed to handle.

Example:

A haircut is done during the time a permanent wave, relaxer, or hair color is processing. The client's name and phone number can also be placed on the appointment screen (Fig. 5–1).

Customer Records

Using a computer, you can access a complete service record with a click of a mouse on a customer name or by typing a telephone number. Some programs require this information to be accessed by the operator's first selecting from the computer's main menu screen, then from a service menu, and then a customer name. How information is retrieved depends on the program, which can be customized by a computer technician.

DAY **Thursday** DATE **6/29** 20 **01**

OPER.	Cathy (STYLIST)	Jacguie (STYLIST)	Mario (STYLIST)	Lucille (STYLIST)	Joy (MANICURE)	Dorothy (WAXING)	OPER.
8:00							8:00
8:15							8:15
8:30							8:30
8:45							8:45
9:00		Carol Gianni cut blowdry 555-1874		Ellen Adnopaz hair color trim 555-2931			9:00
9:15							9:15
9:30	Susan White		Telma Brooks		Kerry Moran basic 555-3396	Abigail Spiegel full leg bikini 555-2940	9:30
9:45	shampoo 555-1561		shampoo 555-5668		basic		9:45
10:00	cut	Linda Klein	set		Sherri Salem		10:00
10:15		braid 555-4166	Catherine Ross	555-9430	tips 555-1647		10:15
10:30	Peggy Neill		cut blowdry 555-8370	Annie Rolland	wraps	Jude Preston	10:30
10:45	hair			shampoo cut 555-9430		full leg 555-6324	10:45
11:00	color 555-9853		Sally McFadden		Lisa Tesar 555-3010		11:00
11:15			perm 555-2993	Jill Brevda 555-8332	basic	Pat Keiler 555-0179	11:15
11:30	Barb Matthews	Heidi Blau		cut blowdry	Nell Sprock 555-0224	lip/brow	11:30
11:45	cut blowdry 555-7207	hair color 555-8129			french	Sue Axelrod	11:45
12:00				Matt Reagan		full leg bikini 555-4012	12:00
12:15				beard trim 555-1300			12:15
12:30	Kyle Harmon		Laura DeFlora		Elisa Klein 555-2817		12:30
12:45	perm 555-1734		perm 555-3276		basic		12:45
1:00	trim	Rich Weller	trim	Ruth Edison	Jim Stein 555-8273	Laura Lowe	1:00
1:15		perm 555-8163		perm 555-2705	basic	bikini 555-5107	1:15
1:30			Claire Sweet	trim	Nancy Goldberg	Denise Carlson 555-4461	1:30
1:45			cut blowdry 555-4278		french 555-1779	arm	1:45
2:00	Allison Nortier			Yolanda Brown		Kendra Miller	2:00
2:15	Shampoo cut 555-0127			cut blowdry 555-2576		full leg 555-2704	2:15
2:30	Jennifer Banks	Liz Collito 555-2703			Linda Douglas		2:30
2:45	hair 555-1320	braid			tips 555-1724		2:45
3:00	color		Liz Daley		wraps	Beth Meadows	3:00
3:15			perm 555-2058	Lori Amsdell		lip/brow 555-7190	3:15
3:30			trim	hair 555-7453		bikini	3:30
3:45	Ginny Chamberlan			color	Brenda Turner		3:45
4:00	Shampoo cut 555-9673				tips 555-0039	Tracy Brost 555-3712	4:00
4:15					wraps	bikini	4:15
4:30	Mary Porter	Anne Thompson		Elaine Zantos		Jasmine Fine	4:30
4:45	cut blowdry 555-2862	perm 555-1117		cut blowdry 555-2873		lip/brow 555-8623	4:45
5:00		trim	Mary Gallagher	Joe Miranda	Shelli Dills 555-4726		5:00
5:15			cut blowdry 555-9612	beard trim 555-4800	french		5:15
5:30			Pam Jeffries				5:30
5:45	Taryn Liebl 555-2878		hair 555-8720		Jacquie Flynn		5:45
6:00	perm		color		tips 555-8047		6:00
6:15					wraps		6:15

Service	Abbreviation
Shampoo and Style	SS
Haircut	HC or X
Permanent Wave	Perm
Electrolysis	Elec
Conditioning	C
Hair Color	HCL
Body Services	BS
Skin Care	SC
Lightening	LTN

Fig. 5–1 Complete service record

Customer Record

Name: Ann Jones

Address: 4675 So Union Street, Morrison, CO

Telephone: (303) 555-1745

Appointment Date	Service	Charge	Operator	Retail Sales
6-17-2001	HC	20.00	Ann	-0-
7-27-2001	HC	20.00	Sue	-0-
8-14-2001	HC	25.00	Ted	6.00 shampoo

Remarks: 8-14-2001—Ann thinks she needs a permanent wave—will call for appt.

Fig. 5–2 Customer record

This screen should be open to all salon personnel. The problem with storing this information on a computer is that *all* salon personnel can have access to it. It allows an operator to have the names and information of all salon clients, and this information can be copied. Unfortunately, an employee can take client information to another salon when the operator terminates employment. With this information, a terminated operator can send out notices on his new employment location, offer special discounts, give premiums, etc., to the entire database of the original salon. Yet, if the salon locks out this information and Ann is absent from work, how is David going to get the hair color formula to serve Mrs. Jones (Fig. 5–2)?

When service is complete, the charge to the customer is recorded on the salon's daily sales record (Fig. 5–3). Automatically, this information is also recorded on the operator's daily records (Fig. 5–4) and on the customer profile screen (Fig. 5–5).

As the salon's operating day progresses, the customer profile screen is accessed and other information is recorded, such as the type of permanent wave given, size of rods used, processing time, operator's name, and results. As this information is recorded by the operator or receptionist, it will automatically access and correct the salon inventory screen.

Salon Daily Service

Date:

Haircut	Permanents	Color	Styling	Total
Totals:				

Fig. 5 3 Salon's daily sales record

Operator's Daily Sales Record Sheet

Name _____   Social Security No. _____

From Week Beginning _____ To _____

Hours Worked _____

Day	Haircut	Perm. Wave	Color	Skin Care/ Makeup	Mani.	Other	Total	Perm.	Daily Sales	Total	Retail Sales
Monday											
Tuesday											
Wednesday											
Thursday											
Friday											
Saturday											
Totals											
Last Year's Totals											

Remarks: ....

....

....

Fig. 5–4 Operator's daily record

Customer Record

Name: **Ann Jones**

Address: **4675 So Union Street, Morrison, CO 80465**

Telephone: **(303) 555-1745**

Appointment Date	Service	Charge	Operator	Retail Sales
1-15-2001	HC	25.00	Ed	-0-

Remarks:

Fig. 5–5 Customer profile screen

As information is programmed on the customer data sheet, production usage can be recorded on the inventory screen. This will give management information to produce the salon's next supply order. The management selects 24 as the desired inventory when all supplies are stocked. At the bottom of the screen will be the quantity to order (Fig. 5–6).

Inventory Sheet	On Hand January 1, 20...	Ordered	Received	Total	Used	On Hand February 1, 20...	Ordered	Received	Total	
Products										*Continued for one year* →
Hair Colors #30	11	12	6	17	9	8	12	12	20	
#32	2	12	12	14	7	7	6	6	13	
#40	5	6	6	11	9	2	12	12	14	
#42	8	12	12	20	12	8	12	10	18	
Perm Waves										
$00.00 Reg.	24			24	12	12				
Tint	15			15	3	12				
Fine	17	6	6	23	8	15				
Spec.	12			12		12				
Higher priced wave										
$00.00 Reg.	10	12	12	22	10	12				
Tint	22			22		22				
Fine	5	24	24	29	17	12				
Spec.	7	24	24	31	21	10				

Want List
Shampoo — 4 dozen
Styling Combs — 14
Natural Bristle Brushes — 10
Hot Combs — 2
Hair Spray — 4 dozen
Hair Clips — 4 dozen each
Rollers — Medium and Small — 2 dozen each
Teasing Combs — 8
Styling Razors — 15

Fig. 5–6 Inventory screen

Operator's Daily Sales Record Sheet

Name   Ed

Social Security No.   000-00-0000

From Week Beginning   1-15-2001   To   1-22-2001

Hours Worked   40

Day	Haircut	Perm. Wave	Color	Skin Care/ Makeup	Mani.	Other	Total	Perm.	Daily Sales	Total	Retail Sales
Monday	25 00										
Tuesday											
Wednesday											
Thursday											
Friday											
Saturday											
Totals											
Last Year's Totals											

Remarks: . . . .

Fig. 5–7 Daily employee sales/salary screen

The computer can also compute the salary of the operator automatically on the *as-service-is-provided* basis. This is done as the operator's sales are recorded.

From the daily employee sales/salary screen the computer can collect information for bimonthly, monthly, and yearly sales and salary reports (Fig. 5–7).

Review of Computer Terms

Hardware. Computer, computer screen (monitor), keyboard, mouse, speakers, printer, and auxiliary equipment.

Software. Computer programs to do specific jobs such as appointment management.

Power. Electrical power from the wall switch or power battery needed to operate the computer. It is best to have each computer on its own electrical outlet with a 30-amp breaker switch or fuse. A power strip with surge protector is a good idea to keep the power source flowing steadily.

Telephone Line

Should a fax or on-line capability be needed, a separate phone line is suggested by all manufacturers for business use. This keeps the salon's telephone open to make appointments.

Computer-Related Problems

The best time to fix a computer problem is before it happens. The following should be considered before you purchase a computer for a salon.

Selecting a Computer Programmer or Specialist In large cities, there are several companies whose sole business is computer programming. It is best not to use friends or relatives because you cannot fire them without the loss of friendship, family problems, and emotional problems. Remember, you are in the driver's seat when hiring a programmer. Tell the programmer exactly what you want. If the programmer cannot produce it, look elsewhere. In large cities, the programmer will probably come to your salon for servicing and training. In small towns, you can use the "eyeball." This is a device that sits on the computer and allows the programmer to view your computer screen as he helps you as if he were sitting next to you. Hint: A hands-free telephone receiver helps when working with a programmer on-line and can be picked up at most telephone or electronic outlets.

Who Runs the Computer? Most salons allow simple programs to be operated by the salon operators—usually this is confined to appointment scheduling and customer records. The training time for these simple programs is two to four hours, and training can be done by the salon owner, a receptionist, or another operator. It is best to select one operator or the receptionist to train the new operator, and pay that person for training the new employee. Don't expect the trainer to do the training for free. But do set objectives for the trainer and pay only after all objectives are met.

The computer programmer should train the salon owner and the receptionist. This should be done when the salon is closed. Several sessions of one hour are more productive than one four- or eight-hour session. The programmer should produce a book or instruction sheet to aid in your salon's education.

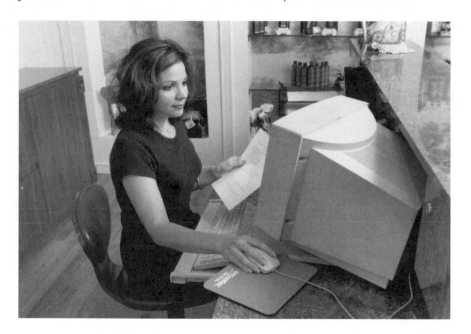

There are usually several ways to perform some of the programmed functions. Computer programmers delight in showing you all the ways to get from A to Z. This inflates the programmer's ego but does more to confuse the student than help. Insist on *just one way* to get the job accomplished. Later, other ways can be taught. Remember when you were learning to do pincurls, and the instructor showed you four ways to do them? After three hours you were so confused you could not do anything. The same is true here. Learn one way. As an owner, you may or may not want the receptionist to do payroll, bank deposits, inventory, etc. Train the receptionist in only those areas that are part of the job description. The complete training program should be taken by the salon owner and another person, such as a husband, wife, daughter, or son, so the salon can continue to work effectively, in the event of the owner's absence due to illness or vacation. As new receptionists are employed, they will have to take the training, and you, as an employer, will be expected to pay for their training and salary during this time. Select your receptionist well. Most receptionists will leave a salon's employment in three to four years.

How Many Computers Does a Salon Need? The receptionist must have a terminal. The salon owner needs a computer in the salon office. The salon system may consist of one computer with one printer, one scanner, or one file server with two keyboards and monitors. Again, this can be designed by your computer specialist. A portable computer (laptop) or a terminal at home with a hookup to the salon's computer could allow some work to be done at home when the salon is closed or when the owner has a day away from the salon. Think ahead. It is best to purchase everything at once so all items work together.

Does the Salon Need Internet Access? This is an item that is helpful for information on products and their use. It can be used for ordering, checking prices, and finding people looking for employment. A lockout may be considered to keep salon personnel from using it for "chat-line" activities or other non–salon-related activities.

Does the Salon Need an E-Mail Address? Generally, this is not necessary. A web page is unnecessary in most cases. A fax capability is most useful when receiving information from supply houses or manufacturers. The question is one of cost vs. usage. If the salon uses the computer to keep track of a chain-salon operation, the answer is "yes." If you have a two-chair operation, consideration of who uses the computer changes.

Handling Special Needs in a Salon

On each screen or computer program a space should be made at the bottom to handle special information that does not occur except once a month or year.

Examples:

When you clean the supply room and discard several bottles of color, this extra space allows you to say "20 bottles of color discarded" on the inventory page. On a slow day for sales the space might read "snow—employees went home."

Cost vs. Benefits

When viewed on a cost vs. benefit scale, each salon must decide on its own as to computer usage. Listed below are considerations:

1. The old paper-and-pen method requires filing cabinets, forms, and space. Computers require less space.
2. In the paper-and-pen method, information is stored in several areas, and files may be difficult to retrieve. Retrieving information should be less time consuming and easier with a computer.
3. The customer records menu can leave the computer and be readily accessed. With the cards system, the cards are sometimes never returned or filed and are often misplaced or taken by the operator.
4. The salon database in the pen-and-paper method may or may not exist. Some salons have permanent wave, hair relaxing, and color cards but may not have names and addresses of hair-cutting clients. With a computer, a database is generated automatically as an appointment is made.
5. If an employee leaves the salon, under the pen-and-paper method, only chemical service cards are available. With a computer, all salon clients are on the database and the list may be copied.
6. The cost of a computer with software, training, wiring, etc., will run from two to five thousand dollars. This translates into a lot of haircuts for a salon.
7. The computer will give you better information, quicker and more accurately. Does the salon need quicker information?
8. A disgruntled employee may destroy or steal a box of chemical record cards but cannot harm personnel records, inventory sheets, etc. However, a computer that is destroyed may result in all salon records being destroyed.

Note: Special "downloading techniques" can prevent this from happening. Consult your computer specialist. However, this downloading or backup takes time, and time is money.

9. The pen-and-paper method has been around for years. The forms seldom change, and pens and paper are cheap. A computer is out-of-date the minute you purchase it. Usually, old software does not work well on a new computer so it is necessary to constantly update.

10. The cost of a computer (complete) may be more than a salon can afford in the short term. A computer that is leased may be the solution. If you don't like the computer or it doesn't function properly you can void the lease. If you own the computer, you may find it hard to sell and recover your money.

The age of the computer has arrived. While small salons will continue with the pen-and-paper method of doing business, this type of business practice will be almost unheard of in ten years. The larger salon will become more and more dependent on the computer, and the owner, receptionist, or a computer operator will control the business information systems by way of the salon's database. As better computer programs are written and developed, operators will use the computer not only for product and customer information but also to show different hairstyles for a customer's facial shape, color, and cosmetic techniques.

Here is some advice on choosing a company:

1. *Reputation:* The company should have a good history within the industry. Talk to others who use that system, and be sure to ask not just about how well the system works but also about how well the company responds when the system *doesn't* work.

2. *Cost-effectiveness:* How will this system help you make money? How will it save you money? These are questions to ask those who have used a particular salon computer system for at least two years.

3. *Operators:* Who will use this computer system in your office? To do what? For the sake of security and to prevent accidental damage (or actual sabotage), limit access to the computer. Be sure the people you choose want to learn the system and are willing to endure a little frustration until they get comfortable with it.

4. *Start with a plan:* Plan the training process (the computer company will help you with this) so that people have ample time to learn. Also allow time for some of the labor-intensive tasks such as typing data into the computer.

5. *Have a backup:* What if the system crashes (fails)? You need a manual system to keep you running while your hardware and software are repaired.

6. *Be assured of quick service response:* Most computer companies offer service through third-party companies that will service your computer on-site,

within 24 hours. Software can often be fixed over the phone via modem. Know the procedures, and have a guaranteed response time in writing before you purchase a system.

7. *Receive upgrades and options at a reasonable price:* When the software is upgraded (improved) how much will the upgrade cost you? It should be a fraction of the cost of the original software. Also, some systems offer options that you can add to the basic package. You save money by purchasing the options "bundled" with the system, but, if you decide to put off buying these, make sure that you can purchase them later at a reasonable price.

8. *Buy a user-friendly package:* Screens crammed with numbered codes will intimidate most users. Opt for a system that is easy to use. Remember that, the faster your staff learns it, the faster you will recoup your investment.

9. *Learn about computers:* You don't have to become a computer whiz, but learning basic terminology and operations before you go shopping will make your task much easier. If you have a friend who uses a computer in his or her business, arrange to spend a few hours learning how it works, or you can take an introductory class at a local computer store or business school. Just be patient. Once you are familiar with the basic terms and concepts, the rest will come more quickly.

Waiting Chairs

These chairs should be attractive and have a certain warmth and charm to them. When purchasing waiting chairs, consider these points:

1. *They should be good looking* and an asset to the decor of the salon.
2. *They should be the correct size.* If your waiting room is small, do not overpower it with overly large waiting chairs. The chairs should be large enough for a 250-pound person but comfortable for a small person as well.
3. *All waiting chairs should be easy to clean.* Be sure that their covering can be cleaned with soap and water.
4. *All waiting chairs should be simple in design* and easy to move around the waiting room. A 2″ × 4″ board, which is covered or painted to match the floor, should be placed behind the chairs. This will prevent a chipped wall, resulting from the banging of the chair against the wall.
5. *Fabric-covered chairs should be long-wearing,* fireproof, and nonporous.

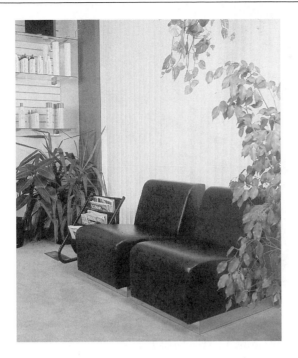

6. *The color* of the waiting chairs should be one of the permanent colors of the salon.
7. *The chairs should have good springs,* padding, and foam rubber. If you cut costs here, you will have to purchase new chairs in three years.
8. *Chairs without arms are more comfortable* because they are less confining and cooler. With chairs that have arms, the air has no way of circulating around the customer.

Floor Coverings

Several floor coverings can be used in a beauty salon. The most popular are tile and carpet. Wood floors, while kind to the feet and legs of the operators, require extensive maintenance. They must be sanded regularly, sealed, stained or varnished, buffed, waxed, and rebuffed. They stain with tints and toners, react to chemicals, and are quite unsatisfactory for the salon business. Besides all the other disadvantages, wooden floors will squeak and warp.

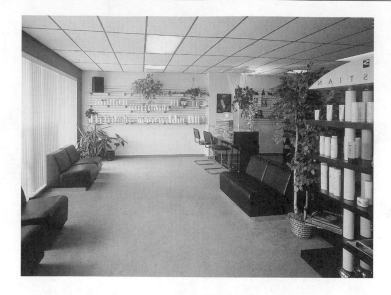

Several types of tile floors are available. Some of these are marble, rubber, cork, ceramic, and asphalt. Marble may be the most beautiful, but it is very expensive. The cost of the marble tile and the installation would bankrupt most salons before they could open their doors. Marble tile will last beyond the duration of the salon. If properly sealed when it is laid, it will not discolor with the use of beauty salon chemicals.

Rubber tile is a good floor covering. The main objection to this type of tile is that it will flatten under pressure. If a heavy person sits in your waiting room, you will notice indentations under the chair legs into the floor. These dents in the floor are the main problem with rubber tile. If a salon has rubber tile, be sure to use an appropriate floor wax. Rubber tile can become very slick.

Cork tile looks good and is fine for a den or a home, but it is too weak to last throughout the years in a beauty salon. Like wood-covered floors, cork tile will stain if not given the proper care.

Ceramic tile floors are close to marble when it comes to standing up to wear. They clean up well and do not need to be constantly polished. The grouting between the tile seems to be the major problem with this type of floor. The grouting placed between the tiles of a ceramic tile floor can discolor over time. If you drop a glass bottle on a ceramic tile floor, it will break. There is no way to cut down on breakage with this kind of floor, but cleanup will be easy.

Asphalt or vinyl tile is now being used in most beauty salons. Its cost is quite reasonable, and it will wear for quite a long time. Also, it is stain-resistant and can usually be polished without becoming slick.

Regardless of what type of floor covering you choose, it should have several important features:

It must be stain-resistant.

It must look good.

It must be easy to match (in case you decide to enlarge the salon and want to use your previously tiled floor).

It should be easy to clean.

It should not be slick when you wax or polish it.

It should be resistant to water spots, crayons, salon chemicals, and wet, muddy shoes.

Carpet can be a real asset. However, some states have restrictive laws concerning carpeting in a beauty salon. Check your state board of cosmetology before you decide to carpet anything other than the waiting room.

Carpeting cuts down noise, keeps chairs from sliding around from place to place, and keeps clients from slipping on freshly waxed floors. It adds a lush look, is almost totally maintenance free, and costs little more than a good tile floor. If you desire to carpet your waiting room or salon, the carpet you select should have the following features.

It should be a short twist or felt type. Long, shaggy carpet will catch on people's heels and cause them to fall. Be sure that the nap is short.

Choose a tweed carpet over a solid color. Solid colors will show every spot, while tweed will hide dirt and other foreign matter.

Pick a light, bright color that will have a stimulating effect on your operators. Dark colors may cause depression and sleepiness. The lighter the color, the larger and lighter the room will look. The darker the color, the smaller and darker the room will appear.

Be sure that the carpet is stain-resistant and can be cleaned quickly. It should resist chocolate, soft drinks, coffee, sugar and cream, bubble gum, candy, and beauty products in general.

It should be easy to vacuum.

It should resist accumulating odors of all kinds.

CHAPTER FIVE SUMMARY

- The reception area is seen first by a client and makes the strongest impression.
- A carefully arranged display window will attract customers. You should take into consideration a number of factors when planning the window.
- Since it makes an important first impression, all aspects of the reception area, from the wall finishing to the computer on the desk, must be carefully planned.

REVIEW QUESTIONS

1. What should appear on the main door of the salon?
2. How often should magazines in the reception area be changed?
3. Who should be responsible for watching children in the reception area?
4. How can you make a room look larger?
5. Why should carpets be short twist or felt type?

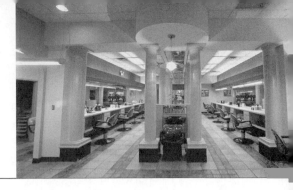

CHAPTER SIX

Decorating and Arranging the Styling Area

Selecting the decor for the styling area is one of the first decisions you will make in your new salon. It should be in the same general style and mood as the reception room (which could be in the same structural area), but, if you should change, be sure that there is a transition area to break the style. The styling area consists of:

- styling chairs
- shampoo bowls
- dryer chairs
- comb-out stations
- booths: for styling, tinting, or special services
- manicuring tables

The way you arrange them will give your salon a definite personality, but be careful that you allow sufficient room to work and that traffic can flow smoothly through your salon.

The Walls

Walls should be easy to clean and maintain. They should be a light color and should be either one of the dominant colors in your decorating scheme or a neutral color. (If your colors are white and gold, then white is one of the dominant colors.

If your colors are blue and green, then white is a neutral color.) You can use any of the colors that tend to make a room larger or smaller, as discussed in Chapter 5.

The washability of the paint used on your walls is of prime importance. A good-quality, long-wearing, washable paint should be used. Due to the amount of hair spray and various chemicals that collect on beauty salon walls, the extra money spent for high-quality paint is well spent. Discuss your needs with a reputable paint dealer, and remember that skimping on this point is not a savings.

The Floor

Floor covering is costly to replace because of the cost of labor and materials and the cost in lost business while the old flooring is being removed and a new one laid. For this reason, choose floor covering that is durable as well as attractive and that does not limit your options for redecorating the rest of your salon.

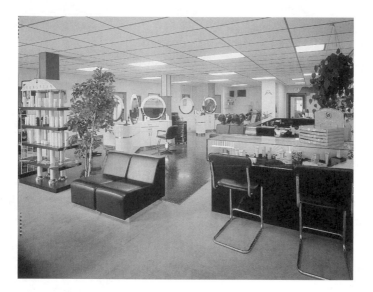

As with other furnishings and design, a floor covering that is predominantly a neutral color works best. Accent colors on accessories can make the salon look stylish and can be replaced inexpensively.

Check the local building codes and your state board for regulations governing what types of floor covering may be used. Choose a type that can handle the heavy traffic without showing the wear and that is resistant to staining and the chemicals used in salons.

The floor should be of a nonporous substance that is easily washable, long wearing, and attractive. Many of the items mentioned about floors in the previous chapter are applicable here. In addition to those mentioned, state board rules must be followed. Some of these rules regulate the use of carpets. Some of the items to check on with your state board are:

1. How close can the salon place carpeting to a wet station?
2. Can carpeting be placed under a styling station where hair is being cut and trimmed?
3. Can carpeting be placed in an area where chemicals (tints, bleaches, and permanents) are used?
4. Can carpeting be placed at a comb-out station if it is used for that purpose only?
5. Can carpeting be placed in the dryer area?
6. What are the fire laws and rules about carpeting?
7. Can electric cords be run across or under the carpeting?
8. What type of cleaning equipment must a salon have to maintain a carpeted area?
9. Are hardwood floors acceptable if washed and waxed?
10. Is a brick floor acceptable if sealed?
11. Are rubber mats, which operators may have at their stations, acceptable?
12. Are throw rugs acceptable for salon use?
13. Are painted cement floors acceptable?
14. Are clay floor tiles acceptable as a floor covering?

Wet Stations

Wet stations are built by companies specializing in beauty salon equipment. Typically, stations are 5 feet per section and are placed on a wall. The sinks are usually in the center and are about 20 inches to 2 feet in width. On each side of the sink there is generally cabinet space. These cabinets hold clean towels, clean combs and brushes, a soiled towel hamper, and a miscellaneous shelf. The top of this cabinet is often used to hold a normal supply of hair-setting preparations for the operator. In back of the sink is the normal place to house the shampoos and conditioners.

Wet stations are ideal for chemical services. Since these are best located separately from the basic styling/cutting station, you can save money on the plumbing

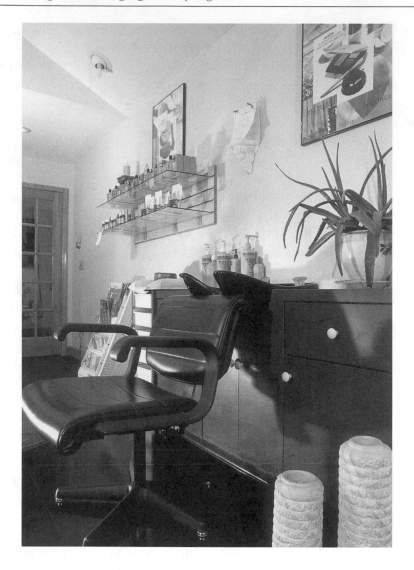

installation by grouping the wet stations and designating these as chemical service stations.

Advantages of a Wet Station:

1. No time is wasted taking the client to and from the shampoo bowl.
2. Once the client is seated, he or she does not have to be moved. This is an important advantage with clients in wheelchairs.

3. Each operator is responsible for the cleanliness of his or her own station as well as restocking supplies (refilling shampoo bottles, etc.).
4. The client can be kept at the sink as long as necessary without interfering with other clients.
5. Shampoo chairs (converted styling chairs) can be raised or lowered to conform to the client.

Disadvantages of a Wet Station:

1. The cost of installation is greater.
2. The styling area is less flexible.
3. Wet stations require more products to be placed on them than a wet area would involve.
4. Wet stations take up more floor space than a dry styling station.
5. Styling chairs are sometimes uncomfortable when in the shampooing position.

The sink portion of the wet station is generally covered when not in use, giving the operator added counter space. When the sink is being used, the top of this section is either lifted or slid to one side, leaving the sink open for use. If the stations are closer than 5 feet (the center of one sink to the center of the second sink), operators will be bumping into one another. The sinks should be from 2½ to 3 feet from the floor. The chairs used for shampooing and styling should be close enough to the sink to let the client's head rest in the sink comfortably.

Mirrors in a wet styling section may or may not extend the length of the station. Regardless of the size of the mirror, it should be kept clean and neat.

Dry Stations or Comb-Out Stations

A dry station can be used as a styling station or a comb-out station. The main difference is that this station does not have a sink in it. While the wet station will extend 7 feet out from the wall (this includes the styling chair), the dry station and styling chair will extend out from the wall no more than 4 feet. The chairs in a dry station should be on a 5-foot center. Placing them closer cramps the operators.

The principal disadvantage in this type of arrangement is that the customer must be moved from the chair to wash or rinse her hair.

The mirrors in a dry station may or may not extend the full length of the

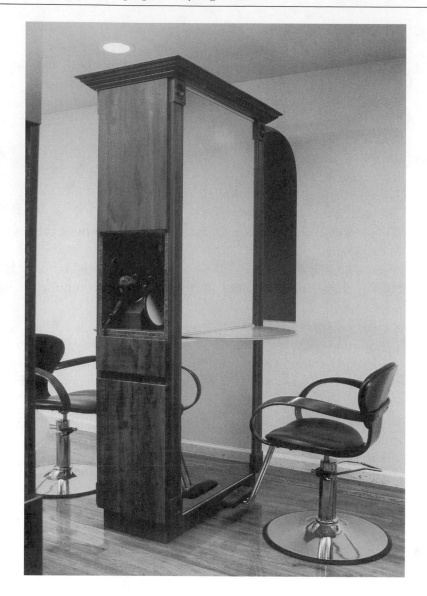

station. They should not extend the full width of the dry station, and they should have a good frame. This will frame the client's face and give a more personal feeling. A growing number of salons are serving both male and female customers. Be sure that the frames on the mirrors of styling stations are not offensive to men. The simpler the better.

Mirrors should be placed so that both short and tall clients can easily see themselves. The difference in height between the average woman and the average man

is about 6 inches. The styling chairs should be able to compensate for this difference in height.

Electrical Outlets on Styling Stations

With current curling iron and air waving methods, additional wiring is needed.
Each station should have electricity to support two curling irons and a 1,600-watt
air dryer. Since some stations are also equipped with ultraviolet sanitizers, clippers,
vibrators, and other electrical equipment, each station should be separately wired.
A good electrical contractor can do this at a reasonable additional cost when the
salon is established; rewiring later may cost as much as four times the original cost.
Put each station on a separate fuse or breaker switch so overloading will not be a
problem. For additional security these switches can be turned off at night, pre-
venting a fire caused by overheated curling irons or faulty appliances left on
overnight.

Styling Chairs

The styling chair is as important to the client as it is to the operator. It should provide full comfort to the client while allowing the operator complete freedom of
movement. If it is to double as a shampoo chair, it should be able to be released
into the shampoo position from either side of the chair. The lock should be easy to
work and should hold securely when the chair is in the lowered position.

All styling chairs (screw type or hydraulic) should be covered in washable,
stain-proof coverings that are easy to keep clean. Chairs with open arms are cooler
and easier to care for than bucket type chairs, and they also prevent pins, combs,
change, and dust from collecting between the sides and bottom. A foot bar or a
foot rest adds to the client's comfort.

Hydraulic chairs should be able to be raised eleven inches with a foot lift. They
should never be placed closer than 5 feet from center to center; to do so would
cause the operators to bump into each other as they work.

Separate release pedals are usually hard to reach with the foot and present
another item to be maintained. Hydraulic fluid and working parts should be easily
accessible for maintenance and repair. Electric hydraulic chairs are not always
worth the extra money. The main disadvantage is the electrical cord, which must
be recessed in order to prevent the operator from stepping on it.

Dryer Chairs

Dryer chairs are usually 2½ feet from the back to the front, including the dryer hood. They are 2 feet wide, and the seats are from 18 to 20 inches from the floor. A footrest may or may not be attached, and this could extend the chair to 4 feet from the back of the dryer to the end of the footrest. These chairs should be the most comfortable in the entire salon. The clients must sit in them for a period of 30 to 45 minutes, and those with long hair may be under the dryer as long as an hour or more.

Dryer chairs and dryers should be like the styling chairs; they should be easy to clean and maintain. The covering of this chair should be of leather, synthetic leather, or a good-quality plastic. Fabrics can be used, but cleaning can be a problem. In most cases the dryer and dryer chair are in one unit, but this doesn't always have to be. The chair can be separate, and the dryer may remain free. Dryers can be attached to the wall or ceiling and, because of their extendable arms, any chair can be used for drying purposes.

A dryer chair should have the following features:

1. It should be comfortable.
2. It should be large enough to seat a heavy person yet small enough to make a small person feel comfortable.
3. It should be able to be cleaned quickly and easily.
4. A footrest, while not necessary, is nice to have.
5. It should place a client in a good position so a manicure can be easily given.
6. It should have a covering that will not cause the client to perspire excessively during the drying period.
7. The chair should have a place to hold a cup of coffee or be designed so that a small table can be brought up to hold one.
8. If the dryer is not attached, the construction of the chair should allow the dryer to be close enough so that the client can sit in comfort.

All dryers, whether connected to the chairs or not, should have the following features:

1. They should come apart easily for quick cleaning.
2. They should be large enough to accept the entire head when hair is set on large rollers.
3. They should be grounded adequately to prevent shocks.

4. They should have a temperature control that is easy to reach by both the client and the operator.

5. One switch should regulate both the heat and fan elements.

6. They should have a re-cleanable filter to filter out dust from the air before it is blown onto the client's hair.

7. The blower should be strong enough to dry the hair but gentle enough not to disturb the hair set.

8. They should be able to be lowered or raised with one hand by either the client or operator.

9. While a timer switch is nice, it can sometimes be more of a hindrance than a help.

10. They should have an automatic cutoff if the dryer gets too hot.

11. They should be attractive.

12. Some salons do most of their business as quick service. This requires hand-held dryers and curling irons. Before investing a good deal of money in standard chair dryers, review the type of service your salon is providing and purchase equipment accordingly.

Manicuring Tables

Manicuring tables are important in the beauty salon. They should be about 2½ feet high and capable of being pushed up to a dryer chair. The height of a manicure table should be such that a patron's arm and hand comfort is maintained during a manicure. These tables should be covered with a nonporous top, preferably Formica or plastic, and should be kept clean at all times. The table should have sufficient light for the operator to give a good manicure. The light should be on the right of the table and should illuminate the working area but should not be strong enough to irritate the patron's eyes. Below the top of the manicuring table should be a drawer to hold the operator's manicuring tools. (Check your state board for regulations covering the care of tools stored in the manicuring drawer.) A stool for the operator should be available. This stool should be able to be raised or lowered as the operator wishes. Casters on the stool and table will allow them to be moved at will by the operator.

Because of health hazards posed by some of the chemicals and materials used in nail services, special precautions must be taken. A separate area for nail stations is by far the best option. The nail stations themselves should each have their own ventilation system to vent noxious fumes and dust outside. Although some nail

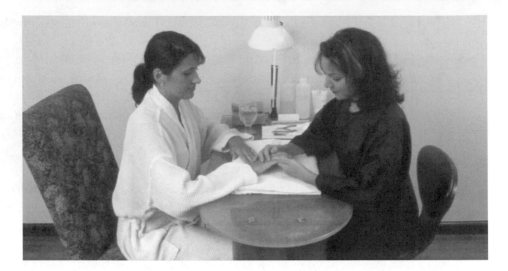

stations have filters and seem to be more advantageous because they require no outside venting, remember that filters quickly lose their effectiveness. Also, some filters remove odors but not the hazard.

You should check with your state board and local environmental authorities to see what precautions are mandated by law, but remember that we live in a litigation-prone society. You may adhere to all regulations and still be sued ten years later by an ill employee because you did not take all precautions that were available—a sobering thought.

Another serious consideration is sterilization of equipment. In part because of the real risk of transmitting potentially fatal diseases and in part because of bad publicity generated by unregulated nail salons that do poor work in unsanitary conditions, manicurists or nail technicians must overcome a negative image. State boards often require basic sterilization procedures. These must be followed scrupulously. Salon owners who want to build their nail business must be sure that the clients are constantly assured that good hygiene is being practiced and that the work is of the highest quality.

Purchasing from a Distributor

Although you can purchase salon equipment and furniture directly from a manufacturer or (used) from another salon, going through a distributor offers certain advantages.

1. The dealer will often give you free help with design in exchange for purchasing equipment from him.
2. Distributors will usually help out with "loaners" when equipment goes bad.
3. Distributors will often pick up defective merchandise rather than your having to make the arrangements to ship it back to the manufacturer.

Coffee

Most salons today serve coffee, tea, or other refreshments to their customers. A clean coffee container along with cups should be part of the equipment in the styling area. If coffee is served, a small table on which to place a cup is needed. Plastic cup holders and plastic-coated cups are quite inexpensive and do a much better job than plain paper cups. Sugar and powdered creamer should also be provided. The coffee container, cream and sugar, cups, and a few spoons should be placed in a convenient place in the styling area for the use of both the clients and the operators. Used cups should be the responsibility of the operator and should be emptied and replaced as soon as possible after use.

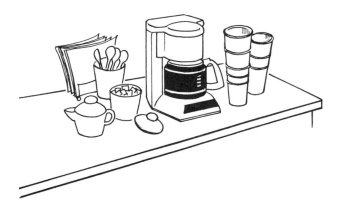

Magazines

These should be the same as those in the waiting area. They should be placed on a rack or table that can be reached by the client. Usually the client will change magazines twice while under the dryer if she is not having a manicure.

CHAPTER SIX SUMMARY

- The styling area should be decorated in the same general style and mood as the reception area.
- Walls should be easy to clean and maintain; floor covering should be durable; both should be of a neutral color.
- Wet stations cost more to install than dry but have several advantages.
- Both styling and dryer chairs should be chosen with the client's comfort in mind.
- Purchasing equipment from a dealer offers certain advantages.

REVIEW QUESTIONS

1. Why should stations be wired separately?
2. What must a styling chair provide?
3. What should be the most comfortable chairs in the salon?
4. Why do manicuring tables need their own ventilation systems?
5. How can distributors help you when equipment goes bad?

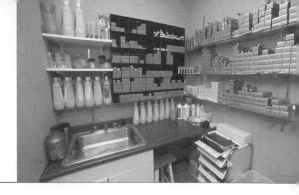

CHAPTER SEVEN

The Supply Room

A well-designed and organized supply room can actually save a salon money. Talk to a salon owner and you will hear, "Supplies are going up." "Our supplies are costing us too much." "I can't make a profit because of our supply bills." A supply salesman once told me that the most costly supplies that a salon can have are those that don't sell and sit on the shelves year after year. How much space you give to your supply room, how you take care of your supply inventory, and how you

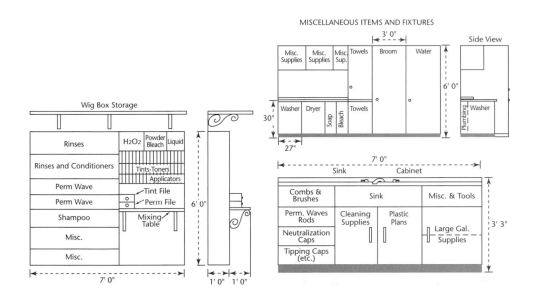

MISCELLANEOUS ITEMS AND FIXTURES

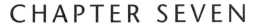

purchase your supplies all have a drastic effect on profits. To get the most from your supply dollar, remember these four rules:

1. Keep an up-to-date inventory on hand at all times.
2. Make and keep a "want list" handy.
3. Place and store merchandise wisely and safely.
4. Take time with your supply agent when placing your order.

Inventory List (or Sheet)

An inventory list is a written account of all the products that your salon has on hand. This list should contain everything: items that are used quickly and reordered (shampoo, permanent waves, tints, toners, bleach, etc.), items that are moderately used and reordered (tweezing wax, antiseptics, disinfectants, shampoo capes, etc.), items that are seldom used and reordered (styling chairback covers, magazine covers, etc.), and items that are not usually considered beauty supplies but are used in the salon (toilet paper, hand soap, coffee cups, etc.). A large book that can be ruled will help in keeping an up-to-date inventory (note the example). Forms and even entire systems for tracking inventory are available from salon educational systems and salon trade magazines and sometimes through a distributor.

You can see from the inventory list exactly how much business you are doing in each of the major areas. This also gives you an accurate check on the number of permanent waves that were bought and sold. If this figure does not agree with your receptionist's desk book, you know that someone is stealing. The inventory sheet is a constant check on the sales and thefts in your salon.

With this book you can make purchasing decisions or you can transfer your information to another sheet and order from it. As your supplies come in, you can use the inventory book as a check sheet to make sure that you have gotten everything you ordered. If changes were made in the supply order by the distributor, the inventory sheet should be corrected.

The "Want List"

This list contains the things to be ordered from the inventory sheet and any other things that your operators might want to order. This list should be posted in the supply room and should be cleared each time that an order is sent in. This "want

Continued for one year ⟶

Inventory Sheet	On Hand January 1, 20 . . .	Ordered	Received	Total	Used	On Hand February 1, 20 . . .	Ordered	Received	Total
Products									
Hair Colors #30	11	12	6	17	9	8	12	12	20
#32	2	12	12	14	7	7	6	6	13
#40	5	6	6	11	9	2	12	12	14
#42	8	12	12	20	12	8	12	10	18
Perm Waves									
$00.00 Reg.	24			24	12	12			
Tint	15			15	3	12			
Fine	17	6	6	23	8	15			
Spec.	12			12		12			
Higher priced wave									
$00.00 Reg.	10	12	12	22	10	12			
Tint	22			22		22			
Fine	5	24	24	29	17	12			
Spec.	7	24	24	31	21	10			

	Want List
	Shampoo — 4 dozen
	Styling Combs — 14
	Natural Bristle Brushes — 10
	Hot Combs — 2
	Hair Spray — 4 dozen
	Hair Clips — 4 dozen each
	Rollers — Medium and Small — 2 dozen each
	Teasing Combs — 8
	Styling Razors — 15

list" will enable operators who are not present in the salon at the time that the supply agent arrives to place their order (note the example provided on page 79).

Computerized Inventory Control

A good salon computer system can be a great help in keeping track of inventory. It will eliminate many of the manual computations, and it can even remind you that you need to reorder. It will not eliminate the need to do a manual inventory at regular intervals so that you can check for shrinkage.

Store Merchandise Wisely

In order to take inventory quickly and efficiently, your supplies should be arranged in an orderly fashion. When you are counting the number of bottles of a weekly rinse, you should not have to look in three places to see if there is a bottle of a certain color.

When new merchandise comes into the salon, be sure that the old merchandise is brought to the front to be used first, otherwise, the unused tints and permanents will be pushed to the rear and will become old and worthless. Since it is hard to get an operator, receptionist, or maid to rotate stock, it is suggested that no supply shelf be more than one foot in depth. It seems that no one minds moving a bottle or two, but moving six or eight bottles is annoying. Be sure to store cosmetics away from heaters and dryers as many types spoil in heat. Keep products away from the sink, unless they are necessary for shampooing.

The Supply Room

The supply room can be as complex or as simple as the owner wishes it to be. The larger the salon, the larger the supply room must be. Several ideas for arrangements are given in words and pictures in this chapter. While no salon can incorporate all of these ideas, they are presented to give you some suggestions on how to improve your supply room. Too often supply rooms are unorganized, and the cabinets are too large. The result is an untidy supply room with no set pattern to it. This leads to wasted products, overlooked products (causing overpurchasing), and wasted time spent by the operator looking for supplies.

Floors. The floor covering should blend with the walls of the styling room and the reception room. Like the floors in these other rooms, it should be easy to clean and maintain. It should be stain- and soil-resistant. Carpeting is a newcomer to the supply room, and it works out quite well. In some cases it has cut down breakage (dropped glass) by as much as 75 percent. A good indoor-outdoor carpet is the best for this room, but any good carpet with a short nap that is stain- and soil-resistant will do. Tile is still the favorite for the supply room. It is easy to clean and polish and is stain- and soil-resistant. Other forms of floor coverings have been tried, but none have been too effective.

Cabinets. How many? What size? How should they be arranged? These are all questions that management must answer. The more operators a salon has, the more space is required for a supply room. A few suggestions follow:

Sink and Cabinet. A double sink is a good idea. A cabinet made of either metal or wood can enclose the sink. A good wooden cabinet lasts longer and looks better than metal. Wood can be painted and repaired and will not rust as a metal cabinet will. Painted metal chips and bends if hit. If you use a metal cabinet, be sure that it is of the highest quality. Stainless steel is not useful for a beauty salon because some salon chemicals react with steel, causing it to discolor.

A good wooden cabinet with a porcelain sink is the best choice. The top of the cabinet should be made of Formica or plastic. The countertop should be molded instead of trimmed. Trimmed cabinets come apart too easily if the Formica comes unglued. If possible, the top of the cabinet should tilt toward the sink for drainage reasons. The cabinet should be at least 3 feet high, 25 inches deep, and from 5 to 7 feet long (note drawing).

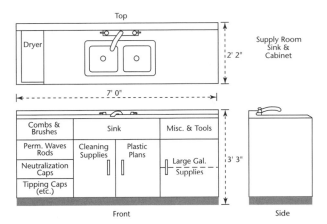

On one side of the sink there should be drawers, and on the other, shelves. Under the sink is a good place to store plastic buckets and any other containers that are used in cleaning. Cleaning materials should also be kept under the sink; these include:

window cleaner
furniture polish
ammonia
sink cleaners
drain cleaners
toilet bowl cleaners
cleaning sponges
cleaning rags, etc.

These cleaning supplies should be placed in a wooden or hard plastic box with handles, as metal will react with some chemicals. Should the sink need repairs, the removal of the cleaning box is quick and simple. Nothing else should go under the sink; this space is not a catchall.

On the side of this cabinet should be a row of drawers. The first should contain brushes and combs that are clean and sanitized and awaiting use. A vapor disinfectant will be needed in this drawer to meet with most state board requirements. The second drawer should contain permanent wave rods. This drawer should be separated into small, box-like divisions. Each rod color should be assigned to one of these boxes. This will make rod selection easy and simple. The third drawer should contain neutralizing capes, shampoo capes, comb-out capes, and, if room permits, plastic capes for five-week rinses. All plastic coverings should be dried and folded before being placed in the drawer as a musty odor will result if they are closed in a drawer while still wet.

The fourth drawer is used for tipping and frosting caps. A heating cap can go in this drawer also. If a manicure heater or manicuring heating gloves are used, they can also go into this drawer. Be sure that electrical cords are placed inside the gloves and cap to prevent a drawer of tangled cords. A manicuring heater can have its cord rolled up and secured with a piece of tape.

Your catchall drawer should be on the other side of the sink. This should contain a screwdriver, hammer, measuring tape, and other items that you need a place for. This drawer must be cleaned at least twice a month. It will house many items that should be thrown out at once and, as a result, the drawer will have a tendency to become extremely messy.

Under the catchall drawer, there should be two shelves. These shelves should be large enough to contain cleaning fluids and the boxed, economy-size supplies for cleaning. Usually there will be several gallon jugs of cleaning fluid, disinfectant, wax, and large boxes of comb and brush cleaner, cleaning compounds, etc.

Supply Wall. A wall covered with shelves is recommended over cabinets (note drawing). The addition of doors to these shelves will cause them to become disorderly and cluttered. When the supplies are standing out in the open, if they look cluttered, someone will straighten them. Open shelves demand attention and stay neat. These shelves should be about a foot wide. They should never be more than a foot deep nor less than 9 inches. If the shelves are deeper, stock clerks will not rotate stock because they have to move too many bottles. If the shelves are less than 9 inches deep a gallon jug will be slightly unstable. The shelves should have a strip of raised trim at the edge to prevent any supplies from falling or rolling off. The shelves should be adjustable in height and anchored well to the wall. Because of the large amount of weight you will be placing on these shelves, they should be well supported and securely attached to an outside wall when possible.

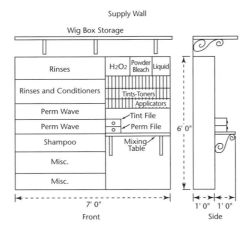

Shelves should be painted with a good oil-based paint and washed frequently. The height and length of such a wall will depend on the size of the supply room and the number of employees you have. Refer to the drawing showing such a wall. Note that shelves start at the floor and extend upward 6 feet. If the ceiling in your supply room is over 7 feet tall, then a shelf larger than the supply shelves (can be 2 feet wide) could be used for the top shelf and could hold things like wig boxes and other light but bulky items that are not in constant use.

A 2-foot shelf, placed 30 inches from the floor, will serve as a mixing table for tints and permanent waves and will serve as an operator's desk. On this table should be the tint and permanent wave file. If the table is used for mixing, it should be covered with a good grade of Formica or plastic. The height of this table should allow a chair to be placed under it.

MSDS Storage

By law, Material Safety Data Sheets (MSDS) must be kept on hand and be easily available. Establish a location for these in your supply room in a folder or notebook. Be sure that the sheets are promptly and neatly filed and that everybody knows where they are and how to read them. Since the OSHA regulations governing MSDS use and storage may change, make sure that you remain up-to-date and make any necessary changes in storage as the need arises.

Miscellaneous Items and Fixtures

Washing Machine

Many salons do their own laundry. If a washing machine is purchased, it should be placed on or against a wall that easily provides water and drain connections. Washing machines are generally from 27 to 30 inches wide and about 30 inches deep, including all connections. The back of the machine, where the connections are located, should be closed off and covered to prevent items from being dropped in back of them. A good brand of machine that is new or just slightly used is best. An inexpensive washing machine may not hold up to daily washings over a long period of time. Commercial washing machines are excellent for this purpose. Many manufacturers offer service contracts that can save you money in the long run.

Dryer

A dryer is necessary if you've already invested in a washing machine. Dryers also are about 27 inches wide and extend into the room about 30 inches. This depth includes installation and exhaust connections. Be sure that the dryer has a lint filter that can be easily cleaned after each load of wash is dried. This cleaning step will cut down on the cost of operation. If the dryer and washer are on an outside wall, you can vent them directly to the outside without much expense.

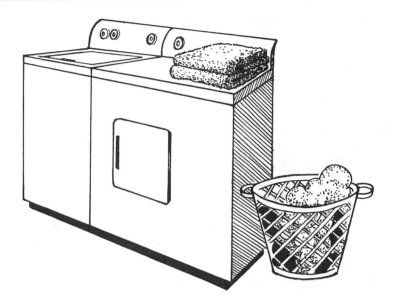

Soap and Bleach Cabinet

The cost of soap and bleach are a major factor in doing your own laundry. A commercial bleach and soap (detergent) can be purchased in 100-pound bags and will produce a savings for the salon. The main problem is where to store the products when you have them. A cabinet the same size as your washing machine or dryer will do nicely. Divide the cabinet in half with two bins. These are usually lined with rustproof metal, but, if made of wood, they should be covered with plastic to protect them from the soap and bleach. The top of this cabinet, if covered with a good Formica or plastic, makes an excellent place to fold the towels and laundry as they come from the dryer.

Towel Storage

A tall cabinet (6 feet or so) should be located next to the soap and bleach cabinet to house the towels and clean laundry. If this is not convenient, a cabinet above the washer will do just as well. The cabinets should be dustproof if possible and kept cleaned and painted at all times. This cabinet should not contain any other items.

MISCELLANEOUS ITEMS AND FIXTURES

Broom Closet

This closet should be at least 3 feet wide and 3 feet deep. It should contain all cleaning implements, such as brooms, mops, scrub pails, and dustpans. A place for each item should be provided. Hang as many of these items on the wall as you can. This will prevent them from being piled into a corner and creating another mess. This closet should have a tile floor, which should be washed weekly. A good rule to follow for the broom closet is "a place for everything, and everything in its place."

Water Heater

This can be housed in a closet of its own or left standing free in the supply room. If it is standing free, it should be washed and dusted at least once a week. The size of the water heater will depend upon the size of the salon and the amount of business you intend to do. Most salons have one water heater; however, two smaller heaters connected in series are not uncommon. This can be done so that, if either heater should burn out, the other one will take over and work alone until the first is replaced or repaired. If you intend to do your own laundry, be sure that you estimate a higher water and electric bill.

Supplies

The amount and types of supplies you use and keep on hand depend on the amount and type of business you do, of course. For example, if your salon specializes in hair color, you will need to stock more hair color products than a salon where hair color is less frequently done. However, state boards often dictate exactly how much of certain items you must keep on hand—usually a specified amount or number per stylist. You can get this information from your state board of cosmetology, but beauty distributors usually keep up with these requirements and will help you stock your salon to meet state board requirements and those of your clients as well.

Take Time with Your Supply Agent

Usually your supply agent arrives at the salon on the same day each week or month. When he or she calls, be sure that you have time to talk to him or her. Your supply agent can advise you on new products and ways in which to purchase merchandise that will save you money. It is amazing how many sales and free merchandise are missed because managers don't take time to talk with the supply agent. Obtain or suggest the salesperson's time schedule, and plan to have all information and orders ready before he or she arrives. This will give you extra time to discuss your needs rather than wasting time searching for purchasing records or "want lists." Use your time with the supply agent wisely, reviewing new merchandise, sales items, promotions, etc.

Retail Supplies

Remember that you are stocking two kinds of supplies: items for use in the salon and those to be sold for home use (retail). A good general rule for determining how much retail to keep in stock is to plan on four of each item per stylist. Thus, if you have eight stylists, you will need thirty-two of each item to be sure that you have enough to handle demand. Of course, if you are assertive about retail sales, you may have to stock more, but money will not be wasted as long as the inventory keeps moving out as fast as it comes in.

Note that each separate item is typically referred to as a "sku" (pronounced "skew," meaning "stock-keeping unit"). If you carry four brands of shampoo, each of which comes in three different formulas according to hair type, you have twelve sku's of shampoo.

Pre-Packs

Much of the confusion surrounding how many of each product to purchase, especially with related products such as hair color, developer, peroxide, etc., has been cleared away by the introduction of manufacturer's pre-packs. These offer the great convenience of a product mix chosen according to the typical use patterns in a salon. Should you need more of one item, you can always order it separately.

Shampoo

Each salon should have a good all-purpose shampoo that is not affected by hard water conditions. This will be used on all clients unless special treatments are required. It should be able to clean the hair and leave it in good condition without stripping tints and toners. It should be a liquid (cream and paste forms are often wasted) and should flow smoothly. The shampoo should be of medium consistency, neither too thick nor too thin. One-half ounce should be sufficient for one application. The container should regulate an even flow of shampoo; too fast a flow wastes shampoo, and too slow a flow frustrates the operator.

In addition to the general use shampoo, the salon should carry a shampoo for dry hair and scalp and one for oily hair and scalp. Shampoos for tinted and bleached hair are unnecessary if the general shampoo is non–color stripping. There are other types of shampoo on the market. Each has its own purpose and good features. But, to supply all shampoos in one salon would be a major financial disaster. If a client really wants a given product, a small quantity should be on hand for him or her, but not for general use. Since a general all-purpose shampoo is to be used in the salon, it can be purchased in quantity at a savings and stored until needed. Be sure to sell that shampoo in your retail section.

Hair Color

Hair color, although one of the most profitable services in the salon, sends shudders of fear through many operators. Because of its complexity, and the very real possibility of a disastrous result if the operator makes a mistake, sales lag. One way you can deal with this fear barrier is to limit your hair color to one line. That way your operators will not be confused by the differences in terminology between one line and the other. Select a line that has strong educational services in your area so you can help your staff overcome their fears and earn more money for themselves and for the business.

As mentioned earlier, the use of pre-packs has greatly simplified the purchase of hair color. In addition to the mix of colors, the pre-pack will contain one each of every volume of hydrogen peroxide. Consult with your distributor sales representative about the available mix of colors and their suitability to your clientele and to the current hair color fashion trends. Ask also about the temporary or semipermanent hair color, as these are a great way of introducing clients to color services and their benefits.

Hair Lighteners (Bleaches)

Hair lighteners come in pre-packs of their own, selected by the manufacturers and distributors to meet the needs of a typical salon. Should you need more of a particular type—oil, liquid, or powder—you can order this through your distributor.

Conditioners

There are three basic types of conditioners. Instant conditioners are real money-makers if used properly and do a wonderful job on the hair if used in a series. The cost is normally small, and one or two different brands of this type of conditioner are recommended. These conditioners usually come in pints. Four to six pints are generally enough to last between supply orders.

Cream or paste conditioners are typically used with the aid of a heat cap. They take longer to apply, and the solution may have to remain on the scalp for ten to thirty minutes. As a result, the cost of this service is higher and the sales are fewer. Two good conditioners of this type are recommended. A liquid conditioner that will treat the hair and remove unwanted casts, spray nets, and other foreign matter comes in pints; one pint will generally last quite a long time. A tube (paste type) of conditioner can do wonders for a client's hair and scalp. A box of twelve tubes provides twelve treatments. Also, the tube-type conditioner can be mixed with other chemicals to improve hair condition following certain harsh treatments.

Styling Aids (Wet)

The number and type of styling aids—lotions, gels, mousses, liquids, sprays, etc.—available can easily overwhelm a salon owner because operators can be extremely selective about which ones they will and will not use. The resulting inventory and ordering problem can add considerable stress to the workday. The best advice to the salon owner is to take the middle road: find a compromise between catering to your operators' every whim and dictating outright which lines you will carry. Remind the operators that, if an operator wants to boost his or her retail income, using products that are sold for home use by the salon will help greatly because this is the best endorsement of a product.

The products you carry will change as new ones become available and as fashions dictate the need for more or less support or more or less natural-looking hair. Be sure to keep a close eye on your stock so that you don't accumulate more of a product than you really need and then get stuck with it when trends make it outdated.

Permanent Waves

Permanent waves are among the more costly supplies that a salon must stock, and sales of these are very vulnerable to the whims of fashion. For this reason, you should monitor how many and what type you keep on hand. You should have four different permanent wave services on your menu, ranging from a budget to a top-of-the-line service. Product price plays a role, but the time and skill involved are the real determinants of service price. You want to have four on hand because most people are comfortable choosing "the high end of the middle." In other words, more clients will choose the second most expensive perm because that signified to them that they are choosing quality without being extravagant.

Hair Strengthening and Relaxing Products

These supplies usually come prepackaged as a unit or are sold separately. Thio and sodium hydroxide products should never be mixed together. While some products are sold in one-pound containers and contain several applications, they must not be held on the shelf for too long a period of time as they may lose their effectiveness. Keeping containers closed will aid in ensuring that the products remain uncontaminated. Some products require a base to be used on the scalp and others do not. Be sure you have all the supplies of the same brand on hand before you start a relaxing process. "A little of this and a little of that" is not the way to operate in this area.

Private Label

Private label products are available through many distributors. These are good-quality products that carry the salon's name on them. You will have to order substantial quantities of these, but the price per item is often lower than for major brands. If your staff stands behind the product, uses it on their clients, and promotes it aggressively, you will benefit from selling private label products in your salon. They also have the advantage of carrying your salon's name on the bottle, constantly reminding your client about your salon.

Additional Supplies

In addition to the basic supplies already mentioned, many other items should be housed in your supply room (for a four-chair salon). Check also with your state board for their requirements.

These include:

1 bottle of tint stain remover
½ gallon of nail polish remover
1 nail polish rack (12-color) and nail polish
1 bottle of formaldehyde tablets
2 cans (2 ounces) of depilatory wax
1 pint of 70 percent alcohol
6 boxes of brush and comb cleanser
1 gallon of disinfectant
1 quart of antiseptic
1 gallon of antiseptic rinse
1 box of cotton in tube form
3 dozen permanent wave end papers
3 dozen neck strips
1 quart of lacquer
4 cans of nail dry
6 bottles (empty)

Standard Equipment

Standard equipment is different from working supplies as it does not need to be replaced as often. It is different from major appliances and furniture as it needs to be replaced several times a year rather than every ten years or so as is true of furniture. Bearing in mind that some of these items might possibly last one or more years, they are:

1 heat cap (for hot oil treatments)
3 curling irons
   small, medium, and large

18 dozen permanent wave rods
  1 dozen very small short rods
  1 dozen small short rods
  1 dozen medium short rods
  1 dozen large short rods
  2 dozen very small rods
  4 dozen small rods
  4 dozen medium rods
  4 dozen large rods

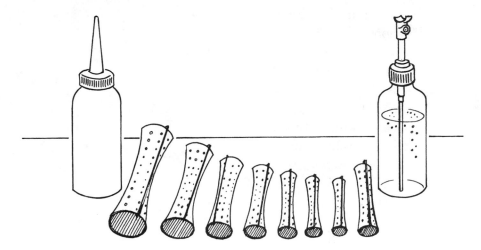

16–20 spray bottles (4–5 per operator)
12 shampoo bottles
6 tint application bottles
6 tint brushes
1 set of plastic bowls
1 set of manicuring tools
12 shampoo capes
12 comb-out capes
4 neck strip holders
1 pound each:
  bronze bobby pins
  black bobby pins
  silver bobby pins

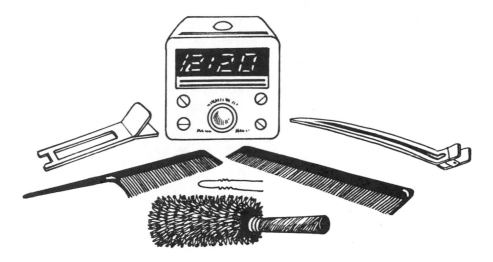

1 pound each:
  bronze hairpins
  black hairpins
  silver hairpins
4 boxes metal hair clips
4 frosting caps
1 package of cotton coil (per operator)
4 sterilizing jars for hair tools (check with state board)
1 sterilizing jar per manicurist
4 bottles of clipper sterilization spray (check with state board)
1 appointment book per operator (often mandated by state boards)
Supplies for artificial nails (vary with brand and technique)
4 electric clippers
4 permanent wave timers
4 dozen brushes (or more)
4 dozen combs (or more)
2 dozen rat-tail combs
1 heater for depilatory wax
1 finger bowl (for manicuring)
4 or 5 boxes of disposable gloves (medium and large)

6 permanent wave neutralizing capes
1 box of large plastic bags (for five-week rinses)
1 brush and comb dryer

Cleaning Supplies

1 broom (straight)
1 push broom
1 dust mop
1 wet mop
1 sponge mop
1 dustpan
1 bottle of window cleaner
1 bottle of furniture polish
1 toilet bowl brush
1 can of toilet bowl cleaner
3 sponges (assorted sizes)
2 bottles of sink cleaner
1 box or can of soap for floor
1 large cleaning bucket
1 large box for cleaning supplies
2 rolls of toilet paper
2 bars of toilet soap
Several rags

Many more items are used in a beauty salon that are not mentioned here. These are partial lists of the supplies you might need.

Towels and Linen

Some salons are purchasing their own towels and linen and doing their own laundry. Other salons prefer to rent linen and have it commercially laundered. If you purchase your own towels, plan on twenty-four per operator. This figure assumes that your salon will be busy. If your salon is new and business is quite slow, a dozen for each operator might be enough. A wise move would be to rent the towels for a month or two and see how many your salon will need. Then you can decide whether to rent your towels and linen or buy them.

CHAPTER SEVEN SUMMARY

- To get the most from your supply dollars: keep an up-to-date inventory, keep a "want list" handy, place and store merchandise wisely, and take time with your supply agent.
- An unorganized supply room leads to wasted and overlooked products and wasted time spent by operators looking for supplies.
- Many salons now do their own laundry and thus need laundry equipment and supplies.
- Need for supplies depends on type and amount of business you do. State boards often dictate how much of certain items you must keep on hand per stylist. Distributors usually keep up with these requirements.

REVIEW QUESTIONS

1. What is an inventory list?
2. Why should supplies be kept out in the open?
3. What does MSDS stand for?
4. What is one of the most costly items a salon must keep on hand?

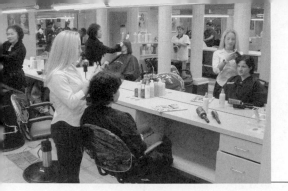

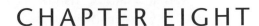

Salon Personnel

After you have selected your salon type, named it, secured the lease agreement, hooked up to public utilities, and selected the decor, equipment, and supplies, your next thought should be selecting and securing a good staff.

The salon industry is experiencing a shortage of staff. The opening of new opportunities for women, coupled with the low earnings typical of many operators, has shrunk the industry's largest labor pool. Good, ambitious operators can now pick where they wish to work.

Salons with mediocre business often have trouble finding new people. Prosperous, progressive salons have more than their fair share of good applicants. Obviously, the lesson here is that, to attract good people, you must operate a good salon to begin with. You must be a leader and a good businessperson.

A note on hiring experienced people: When you hire an operator away from another salon, you have the advantage that the operator brings a good following with him or her. However, if the operator comes to work for you merely because you offered a bigger commission, one of two things will likely happen.

1. You offered too much commission, and keeping this person on staff will not help you make more money, as you are not covering basic overhead.
2. Somebody will offer your operator a better deal, and you will lose your operator and those clients, possibly at the worst possible moment.

To build a dedicated staff you must hire people who are inherently loyal, who appreciate what it takes to build up a business, and who are ambitious enough to work hard. You must work hard for them as well, helping them build their skills and their clientele, and treat them with respect. Even then, there are no guarantees, but you have a better chance of building a strong business staffed by dependable, hard-working people.

Setting Up a Newspaper Advertisement

You may already know one or more operators with whom you wish to build your business. However, most salons must at some point run an ad in the newspaper for securing additional staff to service a growing clientele. Here are a few suggestions for writing the advertisement for an operator.

1. Place the ad in the "Help Wanted, Professional" section. If the first word is either a headline or capitalized, for example, "Hair Stylist," your ad has a better chance of being read by prospective staff people. Obviously, the larger and more elaborate your ad, the more response you can expect. Be sure, however, that your ad matches the possibilities available in your salon.
2. Place the name of the salon in the ad. This gives recognition to the salon and will attract or deter certain classes of operators. (This technique works well in small cities and towns but is less effective in large urban areas.)
3. Place a telephone number in the ad and state "Interviews by Appointment Only." This way you will not be interrupted while working on a client or when you are busy doing something else.
4. State the position (job) clearly, such as, "Hairstylist Wanted, Manicurist Wanted, Receptionist Wanted," etc.
5. The words "experienced" or "with a following" can screen prospective operators before they ever fill out an application form.
6. State the positive aspects of your salon or what you will do for the applicant.

The Interview

When a prospective employee arrives, give him or her an application form to fill out. This gives you the needed data to make a reasonable decision after a few days of interviewing. An example of an application form follows. Without an application form, the interview will wander around in circles, and questions that should be answered will be left unasked. During the interview, use the evaluation sheet to record additional information on the applicant's appearance and personality. A sample of this sheet also follows.

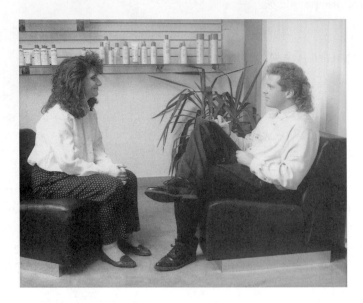

Using both of these sheets will help you to avoid the unwise hiring of undesirable personnel. It costs the average salon more than three thousand dollars in advertising, sales promotion, loss of clientele, and additional salaries before a new operator can make a profit for a salon. Choose your salon personnel wisely.

The information on the application form will help you pinpoint specific areas that you need to explore more fully during the interview. One critical area is longevity on the job. How long does this person typically remain at a job before moving on? If this person has worked at three salons in the area within a few years, you may very well be hiring trouble for yourself.

The questions you ask and how you ask them will help you elicit not just responses but attitudes. Be friendly. Avoid strong reactions to anything the applicant says. Above all, remember that the interview is a time for you to listen.

You want staff who are enthusiastic about clients and who understand that clients can be difficult—very difficult, at times. You want staff who can work constructively with their fellow stylists. Your staff must understand that you, as the owner, are working for them and investing in their future. They should not see you as their foe but as their team captain.

APPLICATION FORM
John Doe's Beauty Salon

Date _____

Name _____

Address _____

Social Security Number _____ Telephone Number _____

Sex _____ Height _____ Weight _____ Property: Rent _____ Own _____

Hair Color: Natural _____ Tinted _____ Bleached _____

How long have you lived in this area? _____ If less than three years,
     state last residence. _____

What position are you applying for? _____

Have you had any experience in that field? _____

Number of years of academic schooling _____

What beauty school did you attend? _____

Do you have a valid, current cosmetology license for this state? _____

Have you ever been a salon owner? _____ If yes, where? _____

Have you ever been a salon manager? _____ If yes, where? _____

Have you ever been a beauty operator? _____ If yes, how many years? _____
     Where did you last work as an operator? _____
     Reason for leaving _____

Have you ever been a receptionist? _____ If yes, where? _____

What salons have you worked at in the last five years? _____
     State name and address of each salon and date of last employment.

1. _____

2. _____

If you are hired as an operator, will you (yes or no):
     Manicure? _____ Permanent wave? _____ Color hair? _____
     Bleach hair? _____ Iron wave? _____ Clean up your own station? _____
     Do cleanup duties assigned? _____ Help on style shows? _____
     Spend one week a year in school for further training? _____

Do you have any hobbies? _____ If yes, name them _____
_____

Do you belong to any clubs or organizations? _____
     Clubs or organizations:

_____
_____

Do you like to do style shows? _____

Have you held any offices in any organizations? _____ If yes, name them

_____
_____
_____

EVALUATION SHEET
(for potential employees)

Name _____

Check the items in each category that seem most appropriate to the interview.

APPEARANCE
_____ neat
_____ well-groomed
_____ appropriate
_____ slovenly
_____ poor
COMMENTS _____

FACIAL EXPRESSION
_____ radiant
_____ thoughtful
_____ sullen
_____ happy
_____ solemn
_____ smiling
COMMENTS _____

HANDS AND FACE
_____ healthy looking
_____ well cared for
_____ heavy makeup
_____ dirty
COMMENTS _____

APPROACH
_____ poised
_____ forward
_____ awkward
_____ alert
_____ timid
COMMENTS _____

ATTITUDE
_____ cooperative
_____ enthusiastic
_____ indifferent
_____ attentive
_____ arbitrary
COMMENTS _____

VOLUME OF VOICE
_____ too loud
_____ easily audible
_____ pleasant
_____ too low
_____ shrill
COMMENTS _____

SPEECH
_____ very clear
_____ pleasant
_____ clear
_____ indistinct
COMMENTS _____

PERSONALITY
_____ magnetic
_____ pleasant
_____ conceited
_____ confident
_____ excitable
_____ animated
_____ tactless
_____ calm
_____ shy
_____ sullen
COMMENTS _____

KNOWLEDGE
_____ clear
_____ understands
_____ uninformed
_____ perceptive
_____ shrewd
_____ ignorant
COMMENTS _____

INTEREST IN POSITION
_____ exceptional
_____ normal
_____ below average
COMMENTS _____

SUMMARY
_____ superior
_____ above average
_____ average
_____ below average

RECOMMEND EMPLOYMENT
1st choice _____   why _____
2nd choice _____   why _____
3rd choice _____   why _____
4th choice _____   why _____
Sorry, don't call us,
we'll call you _____   why _____

One very sure sign of a potentially troublesome employee is the tendency to shift blame from the self to others. Of course, other people do create problems, but a resourceful, positive person assumes some responsibility for his or her own actions and always assumes that there is something he or she can do to improve the situation—without being destructive or hostile. "Bad-mouthing" the former employer or coworkers is a sign of a negative personality.

Here are some open-ended questions that will help you get a look at your prospective employee's attitudes and beliefs.

1. What do you like the best about working in a salon?
2. Describe the best workday you ever had in a salon.
3. What made that day such a good one?
4. Describe the ideal day of work in a salon.
5. What do you find most irritating about being a hairstylist?
6. What is the worst experience you ever had with a client?
7. How did you react?
8. How can such situations be avoided?
9. What makes a good coworker?
10. What makes a bad one?
11. What would you do if you were working next to a stylist who had graduated with you from the same cosmetology school and now earned twice what you did?
12. What are your responsibilities to the salon?
13. What are the salon's responsibilities toward you?
14. What are your responsibilities toward your coworkers?
15. What are their responsibilities toward you?
16. What are your responsibilities toward the clients?
17. What are their responsibilities toward you?
18. How does one solve problems with another person, boss, coworker, or client?

Setting Up a Pay Schedule

How Much Can You Pay an Operator?

This depends on several things. First, is the operator costing you money? This generally is the case when you hire an operator from a beauty school with no following or an operator from another city or state. Second, what are you going to offer the operator as a guaranteed salary? Third, what kind of experience does the operator have?

A new operator, fresh from beauty school with no following, will cost the salon more than $3,000 to get started. This includes the cost of advertising, special sales promotions, and money for guarantees. An experienced hairdresser, without a following, will cost the salon slightly less because he or she will build a following more quickly.

A hairdresser who has worked in the same general area as your salon and has a following will cost the salon very little, if anything. With this type of hairdresser, the salon will run two or three announcements in the local paper, and the expense of his or her new employment ends. You could offer this employee a higher salary and a guarantee.

If you need an operator with a special skill, you might have to spend more money to obtain his or her services. These special skills could be hair color, bleaching, permanent waving, and specialized styling.

If an operator must perform manicures for other operators during his or her workday, you may have to offer her or him a higher guarantee than to those who do not.

What Kind of Salary Will an Operator Want?

It is quite obvious after examining a salon's income statement that only a certain amount can be paid out for wages. An operator who simply wants a place to work, with no benefits of any kind, is now being paid about 50 percent of his or her gross sales. The exact amount will vary depending on the state, city, and location. However, if the operator wishes paid vacations, a high guaranteed salary, health insurance, uniforms, paid parking, and a profit-sharing plan, he or she must be willing to work for 40 or 45 percent of gross sales.

Method of Compensation

There are seven generally accepted ways to pay an employee in a beauty salon. Generally speaking, you should use the simplest possible system in order to simplify your bookkeeping and payroll procedures. At the same time, you want to boost performance by providing meaningful incentives to those operators who work harder and bring in more revenue.

1. *Straight salary.* This is usually reserved for a manager who performs services only when all other operators are busy. If this type of payment is given to

regular operators, it will result in slow work, lack of salesmanship, and a general slowing down of production. In the case of a manager, however, the work involving bookkeeping, bank deposits, ordering supplies, etc., is paid for. If you have a working manager, be sure his or her percentage is the same as his or her operators. A deserving manager-operator can be paid a little extra by means of a salon income override. This override can be a percentage of the salon gross or a percentage of the gross plus an additional percentage of the gross over a stated figure.

2. A *straight percentage* is used by some salons. This guarantee is usually small, and the operator's income normally stems from the percentage of his or her weekly gross sales. The normal way of figuring this type of arrangement is to take the total weekly gross sales figure and multiply it by a percentage figure. The answer is then compared to the given guarantee, and the employee takes the higher figure.

Example:

An operator grosses $650 in a given period. The operator's guaranteed salary is $100, with a percentage rate of 40 percent.

$$\$650 \text{ at } 40\% = \$260.00$$
$$\text{Guarantee} = \$100.00$$

Operator receives a check for $260.00, less taxes.[1]

3. *In some cases supplies are purchased by the operator, and then a percentage is figured as a standard rate.*

Example:

An operator sells two $45.00 permanent waves and has services of $82.00 in a given day. The cost of the permanents to the operator is $5.00 each. The day's salary is figured as such:

Permanent wave is $45.00, less cost ($10.00)	=	$80.00
General work	=	82.00
Total		$162.00
Standard 50%		81.00
Total day's pay		$81.00

---

[1] Some states have laws governing an operator's basic hourly wage. Be sure that the guarantee is over that figure or at least equal to it.

4. *Another way of figuring wages is on a sliding percentage.* Basically it means that after reaching a certain gross sales figure, the percentage increases for the next block of sales. Usually, in the beauty industry, sales blocks are in increments of one hundred dollars. An operator could typically make 40 percent on the first one hundred dollars, 45 percent for the next hundred dollars, 50 percent for the next, etc., up to about 60 percent.

Example:

An operator brings in $850.00 during a pay period, and your salon pays on a sliding percentage—45 percent for the first $300.00, 5 percent more for each $100 after that. The operator's wages would be:

$120.00 for the first $300.00
 $45.00 for the next $100.00 (to $400)
 $50.00 for the next $100.00 (to $500)
 $55.00 for the next $100.00 (to $600)
$150.00 for the rest ($250, the difference between $600 and $850)
$420.00 Total wages

5. *Profit-sharing plan.* This plan is arranged so that all operators, regardless of the time they have worked, receive the same percentage on their gross salary. After a given figure is reached, a certain amount of the profit is turned over to the employees in a profit-sharing program. The percentage of excess profit is determined on an operator's gross total during the period.

Example:

A salon sets a weekly gross of $1,000.00 before they start profit sharing. The profit sharing is at the rate of 10 percent, paid on the gross of each operator. Operator A earns $600.00; Operator B earns $400.00; Operator C earns $200.00.
$1,200.00 less 1,000.00 leaves $200.00 on which the shop will pay on a profit-sharing program; 10 percent of $200.00 will be $20.00.
The profit may be split according to the gross of each operator.

Operator A—gross $600.00—$\frac{6}{12}$ of gross sales or $\frac{1}{2}$
Operator B—gross $400.00—$\frac{4}{12}$ of gross sales or $\frac{1}{3}$
Operator C—gross $200.00—$\frac{2}{12}$ of gross sales or $\frac{1}{6}$

Profit sharing:

    Operator A—½ times $200.00 = $100.00
    Operator B—⅓ times $200.00 = $66.67
    Operator C—⅙ times $200.00 = $33.33

These sums would then be added to the operator's paychecks as an added income for working hard. One thing this system has built into it is a "help your neighbor" arrangement, since what your neighbor makes for the salon may well increase your wages.

The profit-sharing plan described above in no way relates to the *pension-type profit-sharing plan* designed to produce retirement income. With this plan, payment is not paid to the employee but to a fund that is reinvested to produce income.

This money, which is owned by the participant, is put aside without being taxed as income. Furthermore, earnings from this fund are not subject to income tax either.

The monies involved are usually paid out when the employee leaves, dies, or retires. Payout arrangements vary according to how the plan is written. Retirement plans of any sort are of particular interest to those operators who have a long-term perspective and want stability in their lives—very valuable employees. Vesting periods (the time it takes for an employee to earn 100 percent of the employer's contributions to the plan) encourage people to stay until fully vested, at least. However, such plans vary in complexity and appropriateness to your business, and funds can be invested with varying degrees of risk. Consult with a retirement plan expert, and be sure that such a plan appeals to young employees.

6. *A booth rental agreement.* This is a relatively new form of wage and salary idea. Rent is collected by the owner of the salon as either a flat figure or on a percentage of one's gross sales. For this, the owner supplies operators with a place to work. Supplies may or may not be furnished by the salon. A larger percentage of the gross can be paid by the salon to the operators, since the operators are self-employed. Being self-employed, operators must pay their own taxes and insurance and keep their own books. Thus the owner's workload and expenses are reduced, allowing a higher percentage.

The salon owner may or may not be responsible for operators' actions, so liability is sometimes a difficult thing to decide. The salon owner in turn does not have as much bookkeeping and in most cases does not have to pay Social Security or malpractice insurance on renters (in some states the owner will have to). Where there is unemployment insurance to be paid, renters must handle this for themselves.

Example:

Mr. Jones owns a salon. One of his operators rents a booth for $70.00 a week. His operator makes $200.00 in gross sales. Mr. Jones receives $70.00 in the form of rent, and his operator receives $130.00 as a gross profit. Note that no taxes of any kind are deducted. Thus the tax problem and book-keeping now fall on the operator.

A salon owner who enters into a booth rental agreement is little more than a landlord but runs a substantial risk. While free of the need to keep records for the renters, to purchase supplies, and to supervise operations, the opportunity for gain is substantially reduced. Lacking the direction pro-vided by a single owner/manager, the salon's clientele grows haphazardly. Lacking an identity, the salon will have difficulty attracting a particular type of client.

Furthermore, state or federal taxing authorities may decide that the busi-ness is not truly a rental agreement, in which case the owner becomes liable for back taxes and penalties. These can be ruinously high. Abuse of the subcontractor relationship (which is how the government views booth rental) has led to intense scrutiny of any such operation. Because the laws governing this are a patchwork of requirements, some of them painfully vague, the person entering into a booth rental agreement is running a very real risk. And, as many a businessperson has found out, the IRS has author-ity far beyond that of many government agencies, and decisions can seem arbitrary.

7. *Any combination of the other six forms of earnings.* It is possible to mix any of them to get the form of salary structure you wish.

When Should an Operator Take a Vacation?

This is an age-old problem. For new salons it is impossible to know for sure. As years progress, a client traffic pattern starts to form. Salons in one area may have a large number of customers in the summer; others may be busiest in the winter (especially if it is a winter resort). In some areas, farming and harvesting schedules may have a definite effect on traffic flow. Whatever your traffic pattern is, plan vacations around it, and have operators available when you need them. Schedule your vacations during the off season.

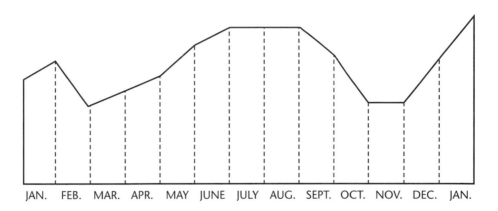

JAN.   FEB.   MAR.   APR.   MAY   JUNE   JULY   AUG.   SEPT.   OCT.   NOV.   DEC.   JAN.

Exceptions must be made; too many, however, will destroy your entire work schedule. Here is a typical business pattern for a salon located in a medium-sized college town near a tourist area. The pattern reflects weekly and monthly volume in graph form, which gives information at a glance.

Note that business volume is concentrated in the months of June, July, and August. This is due to tourist influence in the area.

The drop in October is due to clients paying bills for their children's back-to-school supplies, clothes, shoes, etc. In other words, they are short on cash. Starting December 1st, note the increase in business due to the Christmas holidays. This lasts through January and then drops until Easter (early April). May and September are reasonably good months, due to activities at the university.

With this type of business pattern, operators in this salon should be made to schedule their vacations during the months of October, early November, February, March, and early April. Each salon is different, as is each community. To be able to chart this business pattern, you must keep records over several years.

If you program all your vacations in a row, with each operator taking a week or two at a time, it is possible to hire a new cosmetologist for this block of time. This newcomer, after working a vacation block, can sometimes build enough business to warrant full-time employment. This is a very effective way to bring in new talent without upsetting the rest of the operators in the salon.

Setting Up a Duty List

To keep a salon running smoothly, you must set up a duty list, which assigns certain cleaning duties to each operator and employee. The result of such a list will be a clean and orderly shop. If the saying "many hands make light work" ever applied, it certainly does in keeping a salon looking attractive. The list is important because some operators tend to do more than their share of work, while some will go to any extent to avoid picking up even a soiled towel from their own station. Failure to perform these cleanup duties will cause the cleaning help needless hours of work and lead to loss of profits. Should operators fail to clean up their stations or fail to do their assigned duties, the matter should be immediately discussed. It must be pointed out that failure to clean up leads to extra expense that will be deducted from an operator's salary.

Example:

An operator fails to clean her station and do her assigned duties. A cleaning lady is then forced to spend an hour doing these duties (due to the fact that she is unaware of where things go). The time that the cleaning lady spends should, therefore, be paid for by the operator who made the mess. Her check would then read, "gross salary – taxes, etc. – cleaning expense."

Here are some typical cleaning assignments given to operators in smaller salons having no full-time maid:

1. Operators will wash and dry their own dryer chairs each day.
2. Operators will wash and dry their own styling chairs and styling stations each day.
3. Operators will refill supplies kept at their station at the end of each working day.
4. Operators will clean all combs and brushes they use each day, unless otherwise directed.
5. Clean combs and brushes should be placed at the station at the end of each day (regardless of who does it).
6. Operators should empty their own wastebaskets and wash them at the end of each day.
7. Operators will replace any supplies or equipment taken from the supply room as soon as a service is completed.

8. Operators will be assigned certain duties each day in some area of the salon. These areas should be cleaned up and kept in an orderly fashion.

Your duty is to _____

9. Operators will do their part to keep a designated area in the supply room neat.

Your duty is to keep _____ clean and orderly.

Setting Up a Dress Code and Grooming Policy

Every salon needs a dress code and grooming policy. How an operator looks is particularly important in the salon industry because beauty and fashion are its driving forces. A good general rule to follow is that the employees' appearance should appeal to the clientele. For example, if your clientele is of a conservative, professional nature, the dress code should stress that type of look. Operators can add a personal touch to set off their personality, so long as the entire effect is pleasing.

Uniforms help a salon maintain a standard look. If uniforms will be the rule in your salon, be sure everybody wears them, and be sure that they are distinctively fashionable and adaptable enough to look good on more than a "model-perfect" body.

Uniforms are better if they all match. A two-piece uniform, in most cases, looks better than a one-piece dress. These uniforms should change with the seasons of the year as this will give the operator a lift. Whatever the uniform, its color, style, or shape, it should be clean at all times. A male operator who wears a shirt and tie will not only look more professional but can demand more money.

An operator's jewelry should be simple yet attractive. Female operators should check their slips to make sure they are not hanging below their uniforms. Hose should be clean, and under no conditions should they have runs or holes in them. If necessary, an operator should have an extra pair at the salon.

The hair of an operator should reflect the best workmanship of the salon. All female operators should have their hair done at least once a week in the salon. If the hair is styled in a manner that requires combing, the operator should make arrangements to have this done before her first customer.

Hair coloring should be encouraged, and the cost of such treatments should be paid to the salon. If the salon is selling wigs and hair goods, the operators should be encouraged to wear them at work. These should be sold to operators at cost or slightly below to give added reason for their purchase.

Male employees should wear their hair in a reasonable fashion. It should be clean and neat and reflect good styling. Haircuts should be a twice-a-month requirement.

Makeup should be worn by all operators, but with moderation. A good rule to follow is that "a silent makeup job is better than one that causes attention." False eyelashes and eye makeup should be used in moderation. The overall look should be one of total beauty. If a customer asks an operator, "Where are you going? Your makeup is just beautiful," you can assume that the operator has on too much makeup.

Daily bathing is necessary in our industry. A quick shower before coming to work, with some deodorant, works wonders. If a small amount of cologne is placed at the end of the elbow, a mild fragrance is given off throughout the day. This is pleasing to most clients. Daily teeth brushing is required.

A male operator should shave each day. If a beard is worn, it should be trimmed daily and kept neat.

Shoes should be clean and neat. Be sure that the heels are not run down. Worn heels are especially hard on feet when standing all day. If female operators must have two sets of shoes in the salon, they should be placed in their lockers out of the way and out of sight. At no time should an operator be allowed to work with dirty shoes.

Client Rating of Operators

This takes the form of a letter and questionnaire and gives the salon a constant check on its staff. The letter is general and asks the client for frank answers. The questionnaire does not require the client's signature, and a self-addressed envelope, with postage affixed, will ensure a good response by eliminating costs. The questionnaire should be printed on different colored paper. One color is used for each operator.

To encourage frank responses, assign each of your operators a number, and have the receptionist jot the number and date in a corner of the questionnaire. As the client leaves your salon, the receptionist can hand the client the questionnaire along with a stamped, self-addressed envelope. The client's signature should be optional.

The questionnaire return envelope, when pre-addressed to the salon, should be marked "manager only." This will help you to keep such reports confidential. Better still, use a post office box or home address for this purpose rather than the salon address.

Sample Letter and Questionnaire

Dear Salon Client: _____/_____
                                                        code   date

   Last week you came to our salon for beauty service. We were most pleased to have you and hope you will visit again.

   To help us maintain our high standard of service and better serve you, we ask you to fill out the following questionnaire. Please note that your name does not appear. It is our hope that you will give us frank answers to the questions asked, without fear of hurting the feelings of your operator, stylist, or our receptionist. Please take a minute to fill out this form. You can send it back to us in our self-addressed, stamped envelope. Thank you for your time and cooperation in making our salon better able to serve you.

                                                 Mr. Edward's Beauty Salon

                                                          (Circle Yes or No)

1. Was our receptionist courteous and helpful?   Yes   No

2. Was your operator neat, clean, and courteous?   Yes   No

3. Did your operator please you with his or her work?   Yes   No

4. Did you feel welcome and comfortable while in the salon?   Yes   No

5. Would you recommend your operator to a friend?   Yes   No

6. Did you feel you were appreciated by the operator?   Yes   No

What would you do to improve the salon or its services? _____

_____

_____

_____

   After the questionnaire has been received, the manager should call the operator into the office and discuss results. The information received about one operator is never discussed with another operator. It is noted in the employee's personnel file, which is kept in the manager's office in a locked cabinet. A second or third rating should be made several months later to see if the employee's work has improved or is dropping off.

   A survey every three months should be sufficient to monitor your clients' satisfaction with services performed. A questionnaire can be handed to every client during one week or to every third client over the course of a month. Just be sure that they are handed out in a consistent manner.

Another way of surveying clients is to provide a locked box at the receptionist's desk. Clients can be asked to fill out a survey before they leave and can rest assured that the manager or owner will be the one to read the results at the end of the day or at the end of the week. This saves on postage and will increase the response rate.

CHAPTER EIGHT SUMMARY

- Because of a shortage of potential salon staff, to attract good people you must have a well-run salon.
- Most salons will at some time have to advertise in the newspaper and interview prospective candidates.
- A new operator without a following will cost the salon the most money to get started; an experienced operator with a following will cost the least.
- The seven methods of paying employees in the beauty industry are straight salary, straight percentage, supplies purchased by operator, sliding percentage, profit sharing, booth rental, and a combination of these methods.
- Vacation schedules, a duty list, and dress code and grooming policies should be clearly stated.

REVIEW QUESTIONS

1. How much will it cost a salon to get a new, inexperienced operator started?
2. Who in a salon usually receives a straight salary?
3. What is the purpose of a duty list?
4. What is one advantage of uniforms for the salon?
5. How often should survey forms be given to clients?

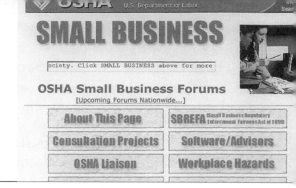

CHAPTER NINE

Labor-Related Laws

As a salon owner you may be or may not be subject to federal, state, and local laws concerning the employment of salon personnel. There are over 400 federal laws pertaining to employees' rights and hiring practices. Couple this with a thousand or more state laws (some relate to one state only) and several thousand local regulations, and you can see the author's problem in discussing this area of salon management in a few pages.

Note: This chapter provides an overview. It is not to be used as a law reference. Consult an attorney in employment law in your state or local community for laws governing your salon's business.

Anyone can bring a lawsuit against any employer for any reason if he or she feels it is justified. Laws are formed in these ways: First, the local, state, or federal legislative structure, meeting in regular or special sessions, can pass a law that governs an industry or special segment of society. These laws may or may not be constitutional but remain in force until challenged. The court system will rule on each law or section of the law as lawsuits surface. This has the effect of confirming the law or defining certain aspects of the law. Laws that have withstood the court action are stronger than those that have not.

The second way a law is formed is by legal action brought by one person against another or a corporation. This is a costly and time-consuming process. When a court renders a judgment, others can use this judgment as a form of legal leverage to settle disputes.

The third way a law is formed is by the vote of the people on an issue. Again, these laws are subject to legal review by the court system and may be found to be constitutional or not constitutional. Each city and township has several "laws" passed by the voters that regulate activities of everything from what is a public nuisance to the activities of business.

Example:

You may not purchase a car or home on Sunday or certain businesses must not be operated in certain areas of the city.

As a salon owner, laws governing the practice of cosmetology and barbering are usually controlled by the state legislators with specific items left to the State Board of Barbers and Cosmetologists to regulate actual practice or activities of the trade. These specific items are known as rules and regulations.

Labor laws do not generally speak to cosmetologists and barbers directly but form guidelines for all businesses to follow.

Labor laws for the most part came out of the 1960s with actions targeted to stop segregation and discrimination. In short, these laws were to give all members of society an equal opportunity for employment regardless of race, color, or ethnic background. Later, the categories of people with disabilities and gender were added. Local communities often went a step further to introduce laws against discrimination because of sexual orientation, age, language, physical handicap, mental handicap, dress, height and weight handicaps, drug and alcohol usage, etc. All this effort was to govern the labor force and its practices.

Usually businesses under five employees are exempt from federal labor laws. The federal government usually deals with laws that are meant to govern businesses with fifteen to twenty-five employees or businesses that conduct business across state boundaries. State laws and local laws may govern as few as one or two employees. Some guidelines are given here with reference material and documents to follow. Remember to consult your labor lawyer to attain specifics in your area.

Guidelines for Owners/Managers

1. Treat all employees equally. A salon document or book given to all employees that spells out hours to be worked, vacation schedules, compensation for work, customer relations, and dress and uniform policies should be the same for all employees. Working hours, evening working hours, cleanup

duties, days off, etc., must be fair to all employees and consistent with the years of service to the salon and related duties. Therefore, a policy book shows that all employees are treated the same regardless of age, sex, sexual orientation, marital status, religion, or nationality and applies to all employees equally.

2. When advertising for a salon position, be sure discriminatory statements are *not* used. "Male only," "must be single female," and "must be under 25 years old" have been outlawed by laws and court rulings.

3. When interviewing be careful of statements you use or the way you state things that might be an advantage or disadvantage to the interviewee. Questions such as, "That is a fine cross you are wearing; do you go to a local church?" and "What does your husband do for living?" do not relate to the job and can have a positive or negative effect on the person obtaining the job.

4. You have a right to have the interviewee take a skill test for the position. However, make sure all applicants are scored on all items required for the job. A male operator must do a facial or manicure if you require all female operators to do a facial and manicure.

5. The compensation (pay and benefits) for the employee must be the same at each level of employment. You may pay employees of ten years with the firm a greater amount than a new hire; however, all employees of the same level must be compensated the same. If you pay Jack more money than Ann because he is a man who is married and supporting a family, you will no doubt be in court soon.

6. The compensation for all employees must be the same, and the benefit package must be the same. However, you may be able to offer different compensation packages if the true value of the compensation is the same.

Example:

$200 each month is awarded as flex dollars. They can be used to purchase health insurance, dental insurance, babysitting services, etc. The main thing is that all employees get $200 in flex dollars, which they can spend as they see fit.

7. All forms of advancement must be the same for all employees. If you offer advance styling classes, they must be offered to all employees. If you send one stylist to a special training seminar, you must send all. You can send them at different times and to different places, but the opportunity must be made available to all and should cost the same amount.

8. Shoptalk is necessary and healthy to promote a good working relationship between employees. However, if the conversation becomes offensive to one individual, it should stop. Female operators who converse about their husband's or boyfriend's physical attributes may offend a male operator, and the conversation could be viewed as sexual harassment. The employer is responsible for making sure no sexual harassment occurs in the salon.

9. A picture of a nude female in a locker may be viewed as offensive to both male and female operators who might be very religious—again, an item of harassment. By the same token, religious beliefs of any nature do not belong in the day-to-day activities of a work environment. Allowing such expressions may have grievous effects if the case goes to court.

10. Keep all employee records confidential and all employee applications and interview forms confidential. All such records and forms are usually required to be held for about one year. Keep them longer, just in case.

Regardless of how hard you try not to break any of the labor relations and employment laws, chances are you are breaking some or bending some without knowing it. Insurance can be purchased to cover the salon owner and management personnel against judgments resulting from a legal suit brought by employees. Avoid at all cost any actions that can be viewed as *deliberate, intentional, willful, or prejudicial* when dealing with one employee over another or one job candidate over another.

For an employee or potential employee to receive damages from a salon or salon management, several items must be proven. All states have different rules, so consult a good labor attorney to see if you have a case. Remember that you may win a court case, but collecting a judgment in the form of cash or compensation may be difficult.

Interview No-No's

All questions asked by the interviewer must be worded the same for each person being interviewed to avoid legal action. Ask only the questions that appear on the interview sheet, and ask all applicants all the questions on the interview sheet, even if you know the applicant or know what the applicant's answer would be. Do not add or modify any questions on the interview sheet. The following two questions illustrate the difference between legal and illegal wording.

Question from sheet (legal): Our salon is quite small and has stations on 4-foot centers. Do you feel working in such a small space would be comfortable to you?

Modified question as asked by the interviewer (illegal): Our salon is quite small and has stations on 4-foot centers. Because you are so large, I do not think you will be able to be comfortable working here, don't you agree?

While some salons are small operations and have under five employees, they still might come under federal and state guidelines for employment practices. This is especially true if the salon is a member of a large national or state chain. The rule here is, "It is better to be safe than sorry."

Major Laws Affecting the Cosmetology Industry

The laws stated here are the major federal laws that have a direct effect on businesses employing over fifteen people or who do business across state borders. Copies can be found in local libraries, from the United States Government Printing Office, and on the World Wide Web. A review of them will give you some insight into labor law.

The Civil Rights Law of 1964

This law deals with discrimination based on race, sex, and religious beliefs. It later was expanded through the Occupational Qualification Act to include age, national origin, disabilities, and marital status. The wording that keeps surfacing throughout the legal literature is that employers must not discriminate when hiring and must make *reasonable accommodations* to support those who are employed. This can be as simple as allowing a person to be absent from work on certain religious holidays. It does not require that the employer pay the wages of a person who is absent unless holidays of other groups are paid. In that case all employees must be treated equally.

The Pregnancy Discrimination Act of 1978

This provides leave time to *pregnant employees or their spouses*. It allows time for female employees to go to and from doctors' appointments, have various medical tests, and take time off for delivery and care of the newborn. The male employee is afforded the same benefit. The reasoning, besides equal treatment under the law, is that he may have to provide transportation, medical assistance, child care, meals, etc., to his wife and children during this time. The employer does not have to provide financial assistance for time lost unless sick leave is requested during this period. The law does not state that the same job, in the same facility, with the same equipment, with the same compensation and scheduling be provided when the employee returns.

Is it the employer's responsibility to provide a time and place to breast-feed the newborn or provide a place to house the infant during working hours? Normally, the answer is no. However, if any employee enjoys these privileges then all have a right.

Since the smells and chemicals found in the salons today might have an adverse effect on newborns, it is best not to have them in the salon.

The Age Discrimination Act of 1978

The Age Discrimination Act of 1978 deals with hiring people over 40 years old. It is fairly straightforward in the beauty and barber trade. If all employees must cut a head of hair in 20 minutes as a requirement of employment, and it takes another employee longer, this may be a reason to eliminate a candidate for a position. The employer is put in a position of having to prove that an employee whose skills are slow due to age is causing loss of income and would put the business in financial trouble. This is extremely difficult to prove because the new employee candidate has no track record for customer service in that salon. When in doubt, don't violate the law.

The salon may not have to consider this problem if the salon is on a booth rental basis for all employees.

The Immigration Reform and Control Act of 1986

This law prohibits the employment of illegal aliens, except under certain conditions. The main issue here is to make sure that the employer has a valid license in the state in which the establishment is located and has legal papers allowing any aliens to have employment within the United States. Should the government question the employment of an individual, the burden of proof falls upon the employer. Thus, copies of all papers for an individual are a must. A good rule of thumb is "when in doubt check first with the Department of Labor within your state."

The Americans with Disabilities Act of 1990

The Americans with Disabilities Act of 1990 and the Rehabilitation Act of 1994 have defined various illnesses or disabilities in a very broad format. While the federal laws deal with operations of fifteen or more people, some state and local laws apply to all businesses regardless of the number of employees.

The new definition of disabilities includes—along with obvious disabilities (loss of limbs, sight, hearing, ability to walk, etc.)—obesity, suicidal tendencies, borderline personalities, post-traumatic stress syndrome, diabetes, and allergies to tobacco and chemicals. Alcoholics and drug addicts are also considered handicapped. To date, thirty states have decided that AIDS is a physical handicap.

The law requires employees to make *reasonable* accommodations to handicapped applicants. This may include ramps for wheelchairs; removal of decorative barriers; purchase of furniture that helps the handicapped; and special equipment such as telephones, lighting fixtures, toilet facilities, etc. However, a situation in which an employee has the ability to generate $40,000 in sales, but accommodating that employee would require remodeling that would cost $100,000 with no guarantee that he or she would stay with the company for a period of time, would probably be found to be excessive.

Employment Contracts

These have been tested in state and local courts across the country. They require a prospective employee to sign a contract in which the applicant agrees to work for a company for a given amount of time for a given compensation equal to or significantly less than other employees. Usually, the decrease in compensation is for advertising, promotions, and education that the salon is willing to provide the new employee. The reason is to give the business a chance to recuperate the cost of hiring a new employee. These costs are usually the cost of advertising, guaranteed wage, training, uniforms, etc. In the contract the new employee agrees not to work for another salon within x number of miles or for a period of time after the employment has ended.

Court cases have favored both the employer and the employee. In cases where the employer has received damages, it was normally for profits from operator's service based on average income generated by the operator until the end of the contract. The salon had to show actual costs of the employee since the start of the contract and those activities directed only to that employee.

Example:

> The employee was paid to go to a training class to further her skills, but no one else was paid to attend a class that year.

If all operators were paid to go to the education class, this cost would not apply. To win this case, the employer's records must be specific to the contracted employee only. The employee, to win this case, must show that the contract kept the person from gaining employment in a reasonable fashion.

Example:

> In a small town of four salons, each of which are less than two miles apart, there is a restriction of a seven-mile radius for working in another salon.

This would eliminate employment in that town and would probably not pass the test. The time limit placed on the individual before employment in another salon is another area of concern. The employee may have agreed not to perform any salon services for a period of two years after this contract in any location except in the business in which the contract is in force. Usually a judge will allow the person to work pending the trial on this contract, which may take up to four years to get in the courtroom. This virtually voids the contract except for the fact that the operator may have to pay for training and other compensation parts of the contract.

Note: The cost of litigation is extremely expensive. The attorneys usually wish to be paid on an "as we go" basis. So you could spend several thousands of dollars in attorney fees, filing fees, recording fees, court fees, etc., and never get any return on your lawsuit. This is true of both the employee and the employer. The time required for these suits to come to trial is also very long. During this time, the operator may have left town, may have gotten married, or may be no longer working, or may be employed in another occupation, all of which will affect the outcome of the trial.

CHAPTER NINE SUMMARY

- Anyone can sue anyone for anything at any time provided he or she feels that some damage has been caused to him or her emotionally, financially, professionally, or physically.

- While labor laws exist, most are designed at the federal level to address businesses of fifteen to twenty-five people or those doing business across state lines.
- More and more communities are adopting laws protecting employees from unfair business practices. Most of these have been based on federal laws but normally relate to businesses of one to fifteen employees or greater.
- While interviewing and conducting business, be sure that the business does not have employees, managers, or owners using practices that could be construed as deliberate, intentional, willful, or prejudicial.
- The Americans with Disabilities Act of 1990 and the Rehabilitation Act of 1994 now form the basis for most labor disputes in regard to employment practices. Before you act, read these laws carefully, especially in regard to the definition of who is considered disabled.
- *Reasonable accommodation* must be followed in making a salon accessible to all employees. The salon should not be held responsible for such accommodations to the extent of extreme financial stress.
- While contracts for employment are used in many areas of employment, those that have been tested have resulted in mixed reviews. These are costly to pursue and usually not worth the effort and time.

REVIEW QUESTIONS

1. What does ADA mean?
2. Name six conditions that might be included in the definition of "disabled."
3. At what three governmental levels can labor laws be found?

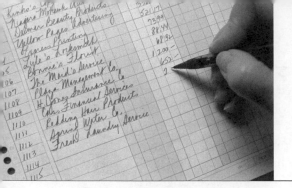

Salon Operating Costs

Salon operating costs will vary according to the salon's location. Whether it is an elite salon or a neighborhood salon, your costs should be held to a certain percentage figure. This figure is based on the salon's gross income. Salon owners agree that profits can run from a low of 6 percent to a high of 20 percent. The reason for this difference is in the definition of profit. If profit means the actual capital gain generated on a capital investment after the bills were paid, then the figures would be more closely aligned. Many owners admit that some of their work is not counted as wages but as profit. Some of the areas where this occurred were maintenance, advertising, accounting, bookkeeping, delivery and pickup, and demonstrations.

Mathematically, a percentage is a ratio of two figures, that is, a fraction created by dividing one figure by a second figure.

Example:

If you have four permanent waves and sell one, you would have three left on your shelf. To find the percentage of permanent waves you have sold, divide the whole or original number into the amount sold. Thus, 4 permanent waves (original amount) divided into 1 permanent wave (amount sold) would be the ratio 1:4 or 1/4; 4/1.00 = .25. This answer multiplied by 100 gives you the answer in percentage terms: $100 \times .25 = 25\%$.

Formula: $\dfrac{\text{Amount sold}}{\text{Original amount}} \times 100 = \%$ of sales

To find the percentage cost of any expense the formula would be:

$$\frac{\text{Actual total cost}}{\text{Actual gross sales}} = \% \text{ of operations}$$

Example:

To find the percentage cost of wages in a salon, take the actual total cost of the workforce in the salon (wages of operators, wages of nonproductive labor, taxes, insurance, records, operators' expenses, and special events) and divide it by gross sales, times 100.

$$\frac{\text{Actual total cost of workforce}}{\text{Gross sales}} \times 100 = \% \text{ wage cost}$$

Keep these formulas in mind when we start to figure projected sales and operation budgets later in the chapter.

Salon Expenses as a Percent of Gross Service Income

Here are some figures that may help in determining the actual expenses of the salon. Usually two figures are given, one high and the other low. Between these figures, any salon should be represented. Profit will be determined by how well you can cut these figures and still maintain the quality of service you wish to give the public. Leading salon trade magazines publish yearly updates on salon operating expenses and profits. You should subscribe to these and compare your own salon's financial profile to that of the typical salon. Remember: You don't want your salon to be average; you want to push for above-average performance.

Wages: 45–55 Percent

Wages should never be more than 55 percent of the gross intake. This figure may seem high, but let us look at what it includes. To exceed 60 percent would cause extreme management problems under present economic conditions.

1. *Wages of operators (productive workers):* These are productive workers who turn out a finished product. They are hairstylists, manicurists, tint and permanent wave specialists, electrolysis experts, and, if you maintain a gift shop, the wages of the person in charge of this area.
2. *Wages of nonproductive labor:* These are employees who do not *directly* produce income. Receptionists, maids, supply girls, shampoo girls, salon

managers (those who do not work on customers themselves), and the repairman (the one who keeps the equipment in working order).

3. *Taxes and licenses*: This is any form of tax paid on an employee. Social security, unemployment insurance, federal taxes, and city "head tax" on workers; all are counted here as part of the wages of the salon to its employees. Include the cost of licenses.

4. *Insurance*: Any insurance paid for employees, on their behalf, must be counted as wages. This includes life and health insurance, retirement income, accident, and malpractice insurance.

5. *Records*: Part of the cost of bookkeeping must be considered as wages due to the fact that the employee is costing the bookkeeper time in making out the payroll.

6. *Operator's expense*: This includes uniforms, vacation pay, tickets to style shows, tickets to workshops, health insurance, and personal advertising in the local newspapers.

7. *Special events*: These are special dinners for employees, holiday gifts, birthday gifts, and any form of bonus paid to an employee for working in the salon.

Supplies: 5–10 Percent

This is a difficult figure to secure, since some salons keep retail items and working supplies under the same heading: "supply costs." Your supply bill should run between 5 and 10 percent of your gross intake. This figure depends to a large extent on how salon products are purchased and the type of product used. To simplify the necessary task of tracking retail sales profitability, separate those items purchased for retail from those purchased for in-salon consumption by your operators.

To cut these costs, distributors have several ways of selling products. Plan to purchase a given item as inexpensively as possible. In some cases, an item must be purchased in quantity and stored to save money.

There are four ways to price a product, which are also the same four ways they are purchased. They are the "each" price, the "list" price, the "deal" price, and the "show" price.

1. *Each price*. The each price is the actual price on a unit of merchandise. Usually this price is high due to the one-unit-at-a-time sale. An example of this would be purchasing one permanent wave at a time.

2. *List price*. The list price is the price on a unit of merchandise where the unit represents several items. Usually the unit consists of 12, 24, 36, 48, or 60 items or more. This will lower the cost due to the fact that only one purchase order is made, one delivery is made, and no odd units of merchandise are left. Usually, this price is about 10 percent less than the each price.

3. *Deal price*. The deal price is usually set by manufacturers to promote sales on a given item. These are specials, and, to obtain them, you must purchase the merchandise during a given period. Usually the period is from two weeks to a month. These items are purchased under the agreement that, if you purchase a given amount, you will get an additional amount free. These free items are what decreases the cost of the item.

Example:

Purchase twenty-four permanent waves at the list price and the company will give you four waves free. When you figure the cost of twenty-eight waves, you can see the savings of the deal price.

4. *Show price*. The show price is usually applied to items sold at a dealer's show. Normally, they will sell an item at list price but will give a certain amount of another item with the show deal. This extra merchandise may or may not be the same as the original item purchased.

Example:

If you purchase two dozen permanent waves at the list price, you will receive fifteen gallons of shampoo free. When you add the cost of the shampoo to the price paid for the waves, you can see your savings. In some cases the show prices and the deal prices are the same.

If you purchase in large quantities and can purchase on deal or show prices, you will automatically cut down your supply bill. To help with the storage problem, some salons have worked out a system in which the distributor will store the item for the salons.

Example:

A salon purchases 240 gallons of shampoo. This is the amount of shampoo used by the salon during a year's operation. The salon purchases the shampoo and pays for it at the show price. The agreement is that the supply house will deliver 20 gallons of shampoo a month to the salon, the remainder to be held at the supply house.

Rent: 5–10 Percent

Each salon has its own rent problems. In some cases it is a flat rent; in others, it is a base figure plus a percentage figure. If a building is being purchased as part of the business, a larger amount of rent can be paid. If the salon owns the building, the rent is actually going toward paying off a mortgage, which becomes an asset to the salon. The average rent paid by a salon should never be over 15 percent, with the best rent being 10 percent.

Included in the rent cost should be the property taxes and the maintenance of items directly related to the building. If you must put an air-conditioning unit in the salon and if it remains when you move, then it should also be figured as rent. Additional figures should be added such as exterior painting, decorating, snow removal, trash collection, etc.

Cleaning and Maintenance: 2.5–4 Percent

Because different salons put different items in this file, it is difficult to give an exact figure. As was noted before, some salon managers and owners do their own cleaning and painting. As a result, nothing will appear in this column. It is quite safe to say that 2½ to 4 percent will cover these expenses. Included in this figure should be cleaning supplies, such as soap and wax for the floor. Other items are brooms, dustpans, mops, polish, and other implements such as small electrical appliances that are used in cleaning. Included as well are toilet paper, paper towels, toilet soap, and air freshener.

Towels and Linens: About 1 Percent

This cost is again dependent upon the salon's bookkeeping system. If the salon does its own laundry, the cost of soap and bleach may appear low. Add to this the cost of the washing machine, dryer, and equipment maintenance, along with the cost of the towels themselves, and costs for towels and linens start to increase. Some salons rent their linens. In this case, there is no equipment cost or repair, and the overall cost is just a percentage of the gross sales.

Utilities: 5 Percent

The cost of utilities is usually about 5 percent of the gross sales. This figure is sometimes included in the rent figures of the salon. This will cover telephone, heat, lights, electricity, water, and gas. Sometimes utilities are considered part of rent costs. If this is the case, this column would not appear.

Advertising and Promotions: 5–10 Percent

The cost of advertising should be between 5 and 10 percent during the first year of operations. Thereafter, the amount should be reduced to between 2 and 4 percent. Tracking the effectiveness of your advertising and promotions will tell you which ones should be dropped and which ones are effective, although you should distinguish between image advertising and promotions designed to bring in business immediately. Utilize direct mail, newspapers, and local magazines, but also think about other, less obvious ways to advertise. Bowling teams, bridge clubs, baseball teams, styling shows, demonstrations, window displays, cabinet displays, and salon decorations all play a great part in advertising and must be considered a part of advertising costs. Radio and television advertising is an excellent way to promote business, but the cost of such advertising is prohibitive for most salons.

Depreciation Cost: 4–6 Percent

Depreciation is governed by tax law. As such, it can vary from time to time. The figure most commonly used is 10 percent of the purchase price. Some small items can be depreciated in one year and are included as supplies. These are clippers, brushes, combs, small appliances, and other small items.

A good accountant should be consulted about the depreciation rate and the current bookkeeping method being used by the government. A good accountant, consulted often, can save the salon a good deal of time and money.

Looking at the table that follows, you can see that a salon that repeatedly spends according to the B column will run in the red, whereas the salon that uses the lower figures in all cases will make a profit of 16½ percent. Note also that in no case do we indicate the manager putting some of his money back into the business. While the figures stated above are standardized, you will find some salons going over and some going under most of these percentages. Cost percentages will also vary in different areas of the country.

Percentage Table*	Salon A	Salon B
Wages	45%	55%
Supplies	5%	10%
Rent	10%	15%
Maintenance	2.5%	4%
Linen	1%	1%
Advertising	5%	10%
Depreciation	10%	10%
Utilities	5%	5%
Total	83.5%	110%
Profit	16.5%	−10%

* As a percentage of gross service income.

Salon Retail Product Sales Expenses

Again, you will find figures for the industry at large in the major salon trade magazines. Compare your performance with that of the rest of the industry, and try to do better.

Cost of Goods Sold: 55–60 Percent

This covers how much you pay for the goods you then resell to your clients. What holds back profitability?

1. *Excess inventory.* Keeping more in stock than you need to. You should never run out, but neither should you have more than a week's supply on hand when your new shipment comes in.
2. *Poor retail sales performance by your staff.* Your staff should average at least 15 percent of their gross service sales in retail. Your promotions should help them sell products, but they must be assertive about sales, too.
3. *Poor buying habits.* If you fail to take advantage of distributors' special show prices or special promotions or, conversely, if you buy items on sale that you cannot sell, you are paying more than you have to for these items.

Supplies: 1–2 Percent

Bags and packaging, especially for such things as holiday gift packages, are a small but important expenditure. Spend the extra money to purchase packages with your salon logo on them; they are excellent advertising.

Invoices and other business supplies should be purchased in six-month to one-year quantities in order to get the best possible price. Again, those with your salon's logo on them are good advertising.

Advertising/Promotion: 2–4 Percent

Nothing sells itself. Clients need to know what's being sold and how it will benefit them. The cost of tent cards, shelf-talkers, and other in-salon signs can be figured in here as well as the cost of samples (an excellent promotional tool) that you give away to build up business.

Commissions: 10–15 Percent

Commissions encourage sales. However, these are not necessarily paid directly to the stylist or receptionist. Many excellent salons put this money into an education fund, which they use to build their staff's skills.

Total Profit: 20–25 Percent

Retail sales profits are an important part of salon income. For example, if profits from retail sales are 25 percent (an attainable figure), and if the percentage of income from retail sales equals 20 percent (also attainable), and your salon brings in $250,000 in service sales a year, the resulting increase in profit to your salon is $12,500 a year. If that sum were invested in a retirement plan for you, you could look forward to an earlier, more comfortable retirement than if you ignored the value of retail sales.

Projecting a Budget

To project a budget using the table above, at least one figure must be known. This projection gives management the number of operators needed and the amount of income that must be projected in order for the business to work on a sound financial basis.

The easiest figure to work with when thinking of opening a salon is rent. As was stated before, rent is usually a flat figure until a certain amount of revenue is reached, and then an overriding percentage may be included. This flat figure is the base on which a salon must operate. Let us now project a budget for a salon.

Example:

Your salon will be located in a shopping center, and you have determined that the typical rent, expressed as a percentage of the gross, for salons in such shopping centers is 10 percent. You know that your salon will occupy 2,100 square feet, and you will be paying $15 per square foot per year. Your rent for the year is $15 × 2,100 = $31,500. Using a mathematical shortcut, you can determine what your salon must gross in order to keep rent costs at 10 percent. You will need to express the percentage as a fraction of 100.

The basic formula for what you have is:

Rent/gross sales = 10/100
Invert the last figure and multiply by the rent to arrive at the gross sales.
Rent × 100/10 = gross sales
Substituting numbers for these, we see that:
$31,500 × 100/10 = $315,000

Now you can easily calculate other costs, using percentages of gross sales based on the national figures, adjusted to your area and situation (you'll have to do a little research). Change the percentages to decimal values and multiply them by the gross sales ($315,000).
Example:

Wages = 52% of $315,000
Wages = .52 × $315,000
Wages = $163,800

Example: Supplies = 5%

Supplies (X)	::	5%
$210,000.00		100%

$$\text{Supplies (X) (100\%) = (5\%) (\$210,000.00)}$$
$$\text{Supplies (X) = \$10,500.00}$$

Completing the table using Salon A, we find

45% Wages	$94,500.00
5% Supplies	10,500.00
10% Rent	21,000.00
2.5% Maintenance	5,250.00
1% Linen	2,100.00
5% Advertising	10,500.00
10% Depreciation	21,000.00
5% Utilities	10,500.00
Total expenses	$175,350.00
Total gross sales	$210,000.00
(–) Total expenses	175,350.00
Gross profit*	$ 34,650.00

* Gross profit is profit before federal, state, or city taxes.
(Licenses are usually considered a tax.)

To check our figures, we go back to the formula

$$\frac{\text{Gross profit (X)}}{\text{Gross sales}} :: \frac{16.5\%}{100\%}$$

Gross profit (X) (100%) = (gross sales) (16.5%)
Gross profit = ($210,000) (16.5%)
Gross profit = $34,650.00

Using Salon B, which has the same gross sales and floor space, and completing the table we have:

55% Wages	$115,500.00
10% Supplies	21,000.00
15% Rent	31,500.00
4% Maintenance	8,400.00
1% Linen	2,100.00
10% Advertising	21,000.00
10% Depreciation	21,000.00
5% Utilities	10,500.00
Total expenses	$231,000.00
Total gross sales	$210,000.00
(–) Total expenses	231,000.00
(–) Gross sales	$ 21,000.00

This gross loss means loss to the company before the payment of any federal, state, or city taxes. (Licenses are usually considered a tax.)

To check our figures we go back to the formula:

$$\frac{\text{Gross loss (X)}}{\text{Gross sales}} \quad :: \quad \frac{-10\%}{100\%}$$

$$\text{Gross loss} = -\$21,000.00$$

Analyzing the two salons, we see certain things remained the same, such as utilities, depreciation, and linen. Since the salon is fixed in a building, the rent cannot be changed. Changes must be made in the expenses of wages, supplies, maintenance, and advertising. While these items can be altered in Salon B, the savings would not result in a profit after taxes large enough to keep the salon operating. This owner would earn a larger profit by putting the money in the bank.

Formula: Number of operators needed equals gross sales per day – sales per hour per operator × hour worked by each operator.

For Salon A

Gross sales per day = $875.00
Sales per hour per operator = 2 × $10 = $20.00
Hours worked by each operator = 8

$$
\begin{aligned}
\text{Number of operators} \ &= \ \frac{\$875.00}{\$20 \times 8} \\
&= \ \frac{\$875.00}{\$160.00} \\
&= \ 5.468 \text{ or } 5.47 \\
&= \ 5\tfrac{1}{2} \text{ operators}
\end{aligned}
$$

You now see that five and a half operators working full-time, eight hours a day, five days a week, will be needed to generate the money to accomplish the goals of Salon A. Unfortunately, this does not take into account the sick days of operators, snow days during the winter months, fluctuation of income at certain times of the year, operators' vacations, or an operator's leaving and moving to a salon down the street. For this, go to the following formula that works well.

Formula: Operators needed as calculated by the steps above + 2. In the case of Salon A, 7½ operators.

Since the floor space of Salon A will comfortably hold only eight to ten stations, you can see the need for securing the right operators (with followings if possible) and keeping your help happy. This was handled in Chapter 8, which discussed salon personnel.

55% Wages	$115,500.00
5% Supplies	10,500.00
15% Rent	31,000.00
2.5% Maintenance	5,250.00
1% Linen	2,100.00
5% Advertising	10,500.00
10% Depreciation	21,000.00
5% Utilities	10,500.00
	$206,850.00
Total gross sales	$210,000.00
(–) Total expenses	$206,850.00
Gross profit	$ 3,150.00

$$\text{Gross profit \%} \quad = \quad \frac{\$3,150.00}{\$210,000.00} \quad = \quad 1.5\%$$

In either Salon A or Salon B the major expense is the wages. Wages must be low enough so a salon can make a reasonable profit yet high enough to attract and maintain good stylists. Many salons have now eliminated the maid, the receptionist, and salon bookkeepers and have reduced benefits such as vacation pay, trade show tickets, uniform requirements, and medical insurance to trim this figure.

Salon A could greatly increase its profitability by decreasing its operating costs and bringing them in line with industry averages. Let's assume that Salon A launches an aggressive cost-cutting effort, finding a more affordable space (lowering rent) and managing its equipment purchases and depreciation more effectively. Let's see how that affects total profitability.

8% Rent	$16,800.00
6% Depreciation	$12,600.00
Total	$29,400.00
Previous rent (15%)	$31,000.00
Previous depreciation (10%)	$21,000.00
Total	$52,000.00
Previous profitability (1.5%)	$3,150.00
New profitability (8.15%)	$25,750.00

Profits from retail product sales should be computed separately, as stated earlier. Assuming the salon makes a 25 percent profit on retail sales, a salon with $210.00 in gross service income that sells even 15 percent of that in retail will bring in an extra $7,875 a year for the salon itself, while operators and the receptionist will receive $31,500 extra, divided among them according to their performance (assuming a 15 percent commission rate, paid directly to the person who makes the sale).

How Many Operators Do I Need?

Looking at the budget for Salon A, the total gross volume you must project is $210,000. The number of days a salon is open a year can be computed by using twenty working days a month using a full staff. Most salons are now open six days a week; however, one operator is usually off each day. Twenty days a month times 12 months equals 240 days a year. Divide 240 by the gross sales per year ($210,000.00), and you arrive at a gross sales volume needed per day ($875.00).

The most stable service is haircutting, and most salons use it as a standard to set prices of other services and time. On the average, a haircut will take about 30 minutes, which includes receiving a customer, selecting the style, shampooing, doing the actual haircut, releasing the customer, making change, and "slip" time (should the customer be late).

Looking at operator service based on haircuts of a half hour each and at a cost of $10 per haircut, each operator could generate $20 per hour. Since Salon A needs to generate $875 a day, you see how many operators must be hired to achieve your goals.

CHAPTER TEN SUMMARY

- Salon profits range from 6 to 12 percent; the range is accounted for by different definitions of profit. If profit were defined as the actual capital gain on investment after the bills are paid, the figures would be closer.
- Salon expenses as a percent of gross income should be wages, 45–55 percent; supplies, 5–10 percent; rent, 5–10 percent; cleaning and maintenance, 2.5–4 percent; towels and linens, 1 percent; utilities, 5 percent; advertising and promotions, 5–10 percent; and depreciation costs, 4–6 percent.

- Retail products sales expense percentages are cost of goods sold, 55–60 percent; supplies, 1–2 percent; advertising/promotion, 2–4 percent; commissions, 10–15 percent; and total profit, 20–25 percent.
- A budget projection gives management the number of operators needed and the amount of income that must be produced in order for the business to work.

REVIEW QUESTIONS

1. Mathematically, what is a percentage?
2. To what does each price refer?
3. How much (as a percentage) of the retail price do salons pay for the goods they resell?
4. What profit do salons usually make on retail goods?
5. What is the major expense in a salon?
6. At $10 a haircut, how much income can one operator generate in an hour from haircuts alone?

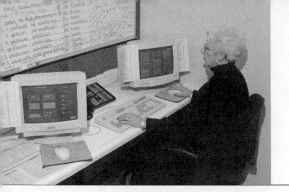

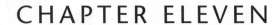

CHAPTER ELEVEN

Salon Forms and Items for Record Keeping

The forms you use in your salon will determine whether you have on hand the information you need to properly run your business. Examples are provided in this book. Salon education companies and trade magazines also sell forms kits and forms you will find useful in operating your salon.

If you decide to use computer-generated forms, be sure you have clean copies on hand in case of computer failure. Keep blank forms in a file marked "originals" so you can photocopy them should the need arise.

Computer software companies have a number of forms used in bookkeeping and other programs. Your computer specialist may wish to copy the forms in this text as a starting point to develop your salon's Management Information System. As you see a need for additional information, the computer specialist may wish to customize these forms to serve your particular salon. Your accountant may also have certain forms he or she wishes you to use or put on your computer. Regardless of how these forms are generated or become part of your computer system, a good rule is to have a hard copy (paper copy) available for review at all times. This is especially true for those records that have a direct effect on the employee's salary. All reports are part of the daily operation of a business and should be kept up to date on a daily basis. See "Management Information Systems (MIS)" in Chapter 5 for additional information.

1. *Employee Application Forms.* A new salon should have some of these on hand. These forms should be stored in the desk file of the receptionist.

2. *Evaluation and Interview Forms.* These, like the application forms, should be ordered in quantities of 100 and should be upgraded as new ones are needed.

3. *Inventory Book.* An inventory book, with all supplies, materials, fixtures, working materials, and all miscellaneous items, should be kept at the receptionist's desk. This book can be purchased from any good stationery house. One book of this type is all that you will need to maintain at a time. A new book should be made each year and should be updated at that time.

4. *Want List.* A pad of paper or a small book to keep a "want list" should be purchased from a stationery supply dealer, and the sheets can be discarded after the supplies have been received.

5. *Client's Appointment Record Cards.* Several hundred of these cards should be purchased at a time as they will be used for each of the salon's clients.

6. *Operator Check Sheets (Client Evaluation Form).* These should be purchased in a variety of colors for identification. One hundred of each color will last a long time. These should be stored at the receptionist's desk, but copies filled in by clients should be restricted to the owner-manager.

7. *Operator's Daily Sales Record Sheet (For One Week).* This form has several useful features. First, it provides the figures needed to compute an operator's weekly earnings. It carries the operator's name and Social Security number, and thus it provides a ready reference.

   The chart itself is divided into several sections relating to each day of the week. If an employee has a day off or is absent from work, a notation can be made for that day. An operator's work is broken down into various activities or services. Note the sample that follows. General work tells of the amount (in dollars and cents) of shampoos, sets, and haircuts that the operator has performed. You might also incorporate the weekly rinses and other small services in this general term.

   Permanent waves, hair color, skin care, and makeup are stated separately in order to track operator performance in those categories. As high-ticket items, these can add significantly to an operator's wages and a salon's profitability, but the management must be able to see how much work is being derived from these in order to give assistance where it is needed.

   "Other" can include special services—hair weaving, for example—not typical of most salons.

Operator's Daily Sales Record Sheet

Name _____   Social Security No. _____

From Week Beginning _____ To _____

Hours Worked _____

Day	Haircut	Perm. Wave	Color	Skin Care/ Makeup	Mani.	Other	Total	Perm.	Daily Sales	Total	Retail Sales
Monday											
Tuesday											
Wednesday											
Thursday											
Friday											
Saturday											
Totals											
Last Year's Totals											

Remarks: ....
....
....

For the sake of simplicity, the salon should pay the same commission on all services. Otherwise, computing payroll can become a bookkeeper's nightmare and can result in increased costs for the salon because more hours must be spent trying to keep the pay record straight.

Additional columns can be added to this sheet as required. These might relate to the time an operator has worked per day and a column for the initials of the operator acknowledging hours worked. When a straight percentage for all work is used to compute an operator's wages, fewer columns will be needed.

8. *Operator's Monthly Report Sheet.* This form states the operator's name and Social Security number and the totals for the month. These totals should be computed at the end of each week and should be a summary of the operator's daily record sheet, which presents weekly totals. (Note example.) Shown in this report are:
   1. The percentage figures that the salon paid to the employee.
   2. The amount that the operator has paid in Social Security, state tax, federal tax, and head tax and any other deductions that the employee might have made. At the end of the year, a yearly summary should be made on each employee. (Note example.)

9. *Operator's Yearly Report Form.* This form is a compilation of each operator's monthly report sheets. These are kept for seven years, just in case there is some question about any of the items. You never know when a government official will want a look at your past records. (Note example.)

10. *Daily Report Form for Salons.* These forms show the entire business operation of the salon each day. (Note example.) It includes the operator's intake, retail sales income, and any other money taken in.

    The right side of the report shows all the "paid out" items. Bank deposits and money shortages are recorded on this side of the page. The report should contain last year's figures and, if a gross difference appears, a written report should explain this under the heading "Remarks." (Note example.)

Example:

On a certain day salon sales were $59.00. Let's say this indicates that the day was slow. Looking at the operator's intake, however, we might see that every operator did an increased amount of business, except one. That operator was absent, which explains why the salon was low in business volume that day.

11. *Weekly Salon Report Form.* Weekly salon report forms are a day-by-day summary of what happened during that week. This information is helpful when

Operator's Monthly Report Sheet

Name . . . . Social Security no. . . . .

January 20 . . . .   Hours worked . . . .

Haircuts . . . .

Perm. waving . . . .

Color . . . .

Skin care/makeup . . . .

Manicure . . . .

Other . . . .

Operator's % . . . .   Operator's wages . . . .

              Total sales ÷ operator's wages = salon cost (%) . . . .

Retail sales . . . .   Operator's (%) . . . .

              Total wages of operator . . . .

Fed. tax $ . . . . Social Security $ . . . . . . State tax $ . . . . . . City tax $ . . . .

Health insurance $ . . . . Stock purchase $ . . . . Wages paid $ . . . .

February 20 . . .   Hours worked . . . .

Haircuts . . . .

Perm. waving . . . .

Color . . . .

Skin care/makeup . . . .

Manicure . . . .

Other . . . .

Operator's % . . . .   Operator's wages . . . .

              Total sales ÷ operator's wages = salon cost (%) . . . .

Retail sales . . . .   Operator's (%) . . . .

              Total wages of operator . . . .

Fed. tax $ . . . . Social Security $ . . . . . . State tax $ . . . . . . City tax $ . . . .

Health insurance $ . . . . Stock purchase $ . . . . Wages paid $ . . . .

NOTE: *By placing a ruler running down the page, you can secure all the figures you need to make out your yearly record. Note that all the federal tax, Social Security, state tax, city tax, health insurance, stock purchased, and wages paid are in a straight line.*

Operator's Yearly Report Form

Year Ending December 20 ....

Name .... Social Security no. ....

Address .... Phone no. ....

City .... State .... Zip code ....

Starting date .... Date of last employment ....

Hours worked ....

Haircut ....

Perm. waving ....

Color ....

Skin care/makeup ....

Manicure ....

Other ....

Total sales ....

Operator's % ....   Operator's wages ....

Total salon cost ....÷ 12 (mths.) = yearly cost (%) ....

Retail ....   Operator's (%) ....

          Operator's gross yearly wages $ ....

Deductions

Fed. tax ....

State tax ....

City tax ....

FICA ....

Health ins. ....

Stock purch. ....

Total ....

         (−) ....

        Total wages paid $ ....

Remarks ....

....

....

Daily Report Form (Salon)

Services Rendered

Operator #1	$ ....
Operator #2	$ ....
Operator #3	$ ....
Operator #4	$ ....
Total services rendered	$ ....

Retail Sales

Shampoo	$ ....
Conditioner	$ ....
Styling aids	$ ....
	$ ....
Specials	$ ....
	$ ....
Total retail sails	$ ....
Misc. sales	$ ....
	$ ....
Total misc. sales	$ ....
Vending machine	$ ....
Total business of the day	$ ....

Bank statement

Cash	$ ....
Checks	$ ....
Coins	$ ....
Total deposit	$ ....
Charges	1. $ ....
	2. $ ....
Total charges	$ ....

Cash Paid Out

1. ....
2. ....
3. ....
4. Refunds
   A. ....
   B. ....
   Reasons: ....
   ....

Total cash paid out $ ....

Bills

	Received	Paid	Held
1.	....	....	....
2.	....	....	....
3.	....	....	....

Cash Report

Total business		$ ....
Currency	(+)	$ ....
Coins	(+)	$ ....
Checks	(+)	$ ....
Total cash		$ ....
+ Total charges		$ ....
Total		$ ....
− Cash to start		$ ....
Total business		$ ....

Long   Short

Last year $ ...... This year $ ....

Remarks: ....
....

Weekly Salon Report Form

Services Rendered by Operators

Monday	. . . .
Tuesday	. . . .
Wednesday	. . . .
Thursday	. . . .
Friday	. . . .
Saturday	. . . .
Total services	$ . . . .

Cash Paid Out

Monday	. . . .
Tuesday	. . . .
Wednesday	. . . .
Thursday	. . . .
Friday	. . . .
Saturday	. . . .
Total cash paid out	$ . . . .

Retail Sales

Monday	. . . .
Tuesday	. . . .
Wednesday	. . . .
Thursday	. . . .
Friday	. . . .
Saturday	. . . .
Total retail sales	$ . . . .

Bills

	Received	Paid	Held
Monday	. . . .	. . . .
Tuesday	. . . .	. . . .
Wednesday	. . . .	. . . .
Thursday	. . . .	. . . .
Friday	. . . .	. . . .
Saturday	. . . .	. . . .
Total bills received	$	. . . . . .

Misc. and Coke Machine Sales

Monday	. . . .
Tuesday	. . . .
Wednesday	. . . .
Thursday	. . . .
Friday	. . . .
Saturday	. . . .
Total misc. and vending machine	$ . . . .
Total gross sales for week	$ . . . .
Balance	$ . . . .

Bank Deposits

Monday	. . . .
Tuesday	. . . .
Wednesday	. . . .
Thursday	. . . .
Friday	. . . .
Saturday	. . . .
Total bank deposits for week	$ . . . .
Total cash paid out	$ . . . .
Total bills paid	$ . . . .
Total	$ . . . .
Balance	$ . . . .

Monthly Salon Report Form

Services Rendered by Operators

1st week	. . . .
2nd week	. . . .
3rd week	. . . .
4th week	. . . .
5th week	. . . .
Total monthly services	$ . . . .

Retail Sales

1st week	. . . .
2nd week	. . . .
3rd week	. . . .
4th week	. . . .
5th week	. . . .
Total monthly retail sales	$ . . . .

Misc. and Vending Machine Sales

1st week	. . . .
2nd week	. . . .
3rd week	. . . .
4th week	. . . .
5th week	. . . .
Total misc. and vending machine sales	$ . . . .
Total sales	$ . . . .
Balance	$ . . . .

Total Cash Paid Out

1st week	. . . .
2nd week	. . . .
3rd week	. . . .
4th week	. . . .
5th week	. . . .
Total cash paid out	$ . . . .

Bills

Received	Paid	Held
1st week	. . . .	. . . .
2nd week	. . . .	. . . .
3rd week	. . . .	. . . .
4th week	. . . .	. . . .
5th week	. . . .	. . . .
Total bills received	$	$ . . . .

Bank Deposits

1st week	. . . .
2nd week	. . . .
3rd week	. . . .
4th week	. . . .
5th week	. . . .
Total monthly deposits	$ . . . .
Total cash paid out	$ . . . .
Total bills received	$ . . . .
Total bills paid	$ . . . .
Bills received but not paid	$ . . . .

Yearly Report on Salon Activities

Year Ending December 20 . . . .

	Gross Operators' Sales	Gross Retail Sales	Misc. and Vending Machines	Special Sales
January	. . . .	. . . .	. . . .	. . . .
February	. . . .	. . . .	. . . .	. . . .
March	. . . .	. . . .	. . . .	. . . .
April	. . . .	. . . .	. . . .	. . . .
May	. . . .	. . . .	. . . .	. . . .
June	. . . .	. . . .	. . . .	. . . .
July	. . . .	. . . .	. . . .	. . . .
August	. . . .	. . . .	. . . .	. . . .
September	. . . .	. . . .	. . . .	. . . .
October	. . . .	. . . .	. . . .	. . . .
November	. . . .	. . . .	. . . .	. . . .
December	. . . .	. . . .	. . . .	. . . .
Totals				

Gross sales from operators' personal supplies $ . . . .

Other sales

1. . . . .
2. . . . .
3. . . . .
4. . . . . $ . . . .

Gross income from 20 . . . . $ . . . .

it is used to chart a graph that will determine operator vacations and planning the supply ordering for the next year. (Note example.)

12. *Monthly Salon Report Form.* Monthly salon report forms provide a summary of weekly operations. They are used to establish bonus figures for each employee when such compensation is involved. It is also a complete summary of what happened in your salon that month. From this you can see if you made a profit for the month or if a special promotional activity has helped your sales over last year. In evaluating monthly figures, be sure that you are looking at base figures. If the price you charge for a shampoo and

Expenses

	Gross Operators' Wages	Supplies	Laundry Expense	Retail Items
January	....	....	....	....
February	....	....	....	....
March	....	....	....	....
April	....	....	....	....
May	....	....	....	....
June	....	....	....	....
July	....	....	....	....
August	....	....	....	....
September	....	....	....	....
October	....	....	....	....
November	....	....	....	....
December	....	....	....	....
Totals				

	Misc. Costs	Federal Tax	State Tax	Local Tax	FICA	Licenses
January	....	....	....	....	....	....
February	....	....	....	....	....	....
March	....	....	....	....	....	....
April	....	....	....	....	....	....
May	....	....	....	....	....	....
June	....	....	....	....	....	....
July	....	....	....	....	....	....
August	....	....	....	....	....	....
September	....	....	....	....	....	....
October	....	....	....	....	....	....
November	....	....	....	....	....	....
December	....	....	....	....	....	....
Totals						

Expenses (Cont.)
Additional Costs

January $ . . . .

. . . .
. . . .
. . . .

February $ . . . .

. . . .
. . . .
. . . .

March $ . . . .

. . . .
. . . .
. . . .

April $ . . . .

. . . .
. . . .
. . . .

May $ . . . .

. . . .
. . . .
. . . .

June $ . . . .

. . . .
. . . .
. . . .

July $ . . . .

. . . .
. . . .
. . . .

August $ . . . .

. . . .
. . . .
. . . .

Expenses (Cont.)
Additional Costs (Cont.)

September $ . . . .

. . . .

. . . .

. . . .

October $ . . . .

. . . .

. . . .

. . . .

November $ . . . .

. . . .

. . . .

. . . .

December $ . . . .

. . . .

. . . .

. . . .

                                    Total additional cost $ . . . .

Total operators' wages	$	Total federal tax	$ . . . .
Total supply cost	$	Total state tax	$ . . . .
Total laundry expense	$	Total FICA	$ . . . .
Total retail items cost	$	Total licenses	$ . . . .
Total additional cost	$	Total misc. cost	$ . . . .
Total yearly expenses	$		
Gross Income for 20 . . .	$		
Yearly expenses (–)	$		
Gross profit	$		

Cost of money
   (interest on principal from bank mortgage) $ . . . .

Money paid on principal $ . . . .

                                    Total $ . . . .

Net profit (gross profit – money cost and principal payment) $ . . . .

Expenses Cont.

Remarks:

· ·

· ·

· ·

· ·

Future Operation Plans:

· ·

· ·

· ·

· ·

---

set has gone up during the year, the base figure could be different. (Note example.)

Example:

Comparing figures shows that the salon made an increase in sales this year of 8 percent. On the surface this looks good. If, however, you raised prices 12 percent over the past year, you are actually running behind last year in business volume.

13. *Yearly Report on Salon Activities.* After you have the twelve monthly salon report forms completed, you will find little trouble figuring taxes, wages, profits, and cost. From this information you should compile and write a yearly report. In this report you should state your profit, what you lost money on, amounts you paid out in all areas, and, most important, what you intend to do in the future. This is important because it establishes, in writing, a direction for your salon. Furthermore, if you should sell, die, or become unable to run the salon, the person who takes your place knows where you have been and where you are heading. Your accountant may also find it helpful when counseling you on finance.

14. *Bank Deposit Record Book.* This is a book in which all deposits are recorded by the bank. It is given to the salon by the bank, and each day, as deposits are made, they are recorded. The deposit book contains the account number, the date of transaction, and the initials of the teller who takes the deposit.

This book then becomes a ready reference for the amount you have in the bank. The amount of each deposit should be entered immediately in the computer accounting files in order to avoid mistakes. If you use an automatic teller machine, be sure to keep the record of the transaction until the deposit is recorded on your next statement.

An example:

An example: Account Number 70-2345		
Date	Amount	Teller
4-1-20__	$250.00	J. W.
4-2-20__	$323.00	B. V.
4-3-20__	$274.25	J. R.

15. *Bank Deposit Receipts*. Deposit receipts are a receipt for the money you have deposited at the bank. They should show the same amount that the salon grossed the day before (the charges). These receipts should be stapled to the daily salon report and filed away with it.

16. *Checkbook*. This book of checks is for salon use only. Any check written on this account should be for a business expense. Personal checks written on business accounts cause tax problems and pave the way to a bankrupt salon. The checkbook comes in several forms, with several types of information stubs. Your banker will help you select the proper type for your particular business.

17. *Employees' Tip Report Form*. This form can be obtained by writing your local Internal Revenue Service office. These forms are given to all employees. Employees are required to state the amount of tips over a specified figure and return the form to you. You are required to withhold taxes on that amount from their regular salary checks. This is a safeguard for the operator, so he or she will not end the year owing the government additional income tax.

18. *Tax Forms*.[1] Forms for collecting and remitting tax money can be obtained

---

[1] If an accountant is doing your bookkeeping, he or she will have these forms and all related information available in his or her office. A good accountant can save the salon time, effort, energy, and money because of his or her knowledge of the tax structure and tax requirements.

free from any Internal Revenue Service office. In some cases you will have three or more forms to fill out and send: one for the federal government, one for the state government, one for city head tax, or income tax. State sales tax, federal sales tax, and taxes on vending machines may all have to be remitted. Forms for each of these should accompany your salon's tax payment check.

19. *Operators' Tally Sheets*. These usually take the form of printed tickets. They consist of the operator's name, the customer's name, the service rendered, the date, and the cost of the service. The customer will regard this as his or her bill and will pay the total amount at the receptionist's desk. The tally remains the property of the salon, regardless of how the customer pays the bill. Keep tally sheets, sales tickets, and/or the computer records of these for the time prescribed by law, seven years, as they are important tax records of operators' services rendered and appointments kept. If there is a question about the amount of business done on a given day by an operator, all that is needed to answer the question is to add the tallies of that particular operator. Tickets should be numbered so that extra tickets cannot be added or subtracted. If your salon accepts credit cards, the client will receive one copy. The others are for your own records and to send to the credit card company for their own records and billing purposes.

20. *Appointment Cards*. These are cards that confirm a salon appointment. Several things have to be included on these cards. First, they should have the salon's name, address, and telephone number. Next, they should have a space for the time, service, and the operator's name. A small note at the bottom of the card stating "If an appointment is not canceled at least twenty-four hours before the time of appointment, a charge will be made" has been an effective means of discouraging customers from not showing up as scheduled. Whether you will actually attempt to collect will depend on your working relationship and respect for the customer. An appointment card is shown on the next page as an example.

21. *Appointment Book*. This is the most important record in your salon. Be sure that this book is large enough to handle all operators in your salon. It should be bound with a hard cover, as it will be filed away as a permanent record of the salon's activities.

   Some salon computer systems have appointment books. These should be saved at the end of each day for income tax purposes. The information on all appointments for the next day should be printed out at the close of business the night before and backed up regularly in order to prevent a disaster. Remember that your computer system will eventually crash. If you have the

Appointment Card

Salon's Name . . . .

Address . . . .

Telephone No. . . . .

Time . . . .   Service . . . .

Operator's Name . . . .

If an appointment is not canceled at least twenty-four hours before the time of appointment, a charge will be made.

data backed up, the crash will mean a short-term headache. If you don't have data backed up, you will never forget the day it happened—or the weeks that followed.

The appointment book should have a column for each operator. Once operators have placed their name in the book, their column should never be changed. The reason for this is that operators and receptionists tend to form the habit of looking at a given column for information concerning a particular operator instead of checking to see if it's the right name.

It will take about three weeks for a new habit to be learned if names are rearranged in the appointment book. During this time, your salon will be in a complete state of disaster as far as the appointment book is concerned.

The time of the day is an important part of an appointment book and should be boxed off with dark lines for hours and spaced on the fifteen-minute marks.

Example:

   10:00
   10:15
   10:30
   10:45
   11:00

When a person calls for an appointment, his or her name should be recorded in pencil. If the appointment is later canceled, you can easily erase it. The appropriate time should be on the book for the service, and the type of service should be stated. In most cases, the service will be stated in an abbreviated form. Some of

DAY __Thursday_____ DATE _____6/29_____ 20_01_____

OPER.	Cathy (STYLIST)	Jacquie (STYLIST)	Mario (STYLIST)	Lucille (STYLIST)	Joy (MANICURE)	Dorothy (WAXING)	OPER.
8:00							8:00
8:15							8:15
8:30							8:30
8:45							8:45
9:00		Carol Gianni		Ellen Adnopaz			9:00
9:15		cut blowdry 555-1874		hair color trim 555-2931			9:15
9:30	Susan White		Telma Brooks		Kerry Moran	Abigail Spiegel	9:30
9:45	shampoo 555-1561		shampoo 555-5668		basic 555-3396	full leg bikini 555-2940	9:45
10:00	cut	Linda Klein	set		Sherri Salem		10:00
10:15		braid 555-4166	Catherine Ross	555-9430	tips 555-1647		10:15
10:30	Peggy Neill		cut blowdry 555-8370	Annie Rolland	wraps	Jude Preston	10:30
10:45	hair 555-9853			shampoo cut 555-9430		full leg 555-6324	10:45
11:00	color		Sally McFadden		Lisa Tesar 555-		11:00
11:15			perm 555-2993	Jill Brevda	basic 3010	Pat Keiler 555-	11:15
11:30	Barb Matthews	Heidi Blau		cut blowdry 555-8332	Nell Sprock 555-	lip/brow 0179	11:30
11:45	cut blowdry 555-7207	hair color 555-8129			french 0224	Sue Axelrod	11:45
12:00				Matt Reagan		full leg 555-4012	12:00
12:15				beard trim 555-1300		bikini	12:15
12:30	Kyle Harmon		Laura Deflora		Elisa Klein 555-		12:30
12:45	perm 555-1734		perm 555-3276		basic 2817		12:45
1:00	trim	Rich Weller	trim	Ruth Edison	Jim Stein 555-	Laura Lowe	1:00
1:15		perm 555-8163		perm 555-2705	basic 8273	bikini 555-5107	1:15
1:30			Claire Sweet	trim	Nancy Goldberg	Denise Carlson	1:30
1:45			cut blowdry 555-4278		french 555-1779	arm 555-4461	1:45
2:00	Allison Nortier			Yolanda Brown		Kendra Miller	2:00
2:15	shampoo cut 555-0127			cut blowdry 555-2576		full leg 555-2704	2:15
2:30	Jennifer Banks	Liz Collito			Linda Douglas		2:30
2:45	hair 555-1320	braid 555-2703			tips 555-1724		2:45
3:00	color		Liz Daley		wraps	Beth Meadows	3:00
3:15			perm 555-2058	Lori Amsdell		lip/brow 555-7190	3:15
3:30			trim	hair 555-7453		bikini	3:30
3:45	Ginny Chamberlan			color	Brenda Turner		3:45
4:00	shampoo cut 555-9673				tips 555-0039	Tracy Brost 555-	4:00
4:15					wraps	bikini 3712	4:15
4:30	Mary Porter	Anne Thompson		Elaine Zantos		Jasmine Fine	4:30
4:45	cut blowdry 555-2862	perm 555-1117		cut blowdry 2873		lip/brow 555-8623	4:45
5:00		trim	Mary Gallagher	Joe Miranda	Shelli Dills		5:00
5:15			cut blowdry 555-9612	beard trim 555-4800	french 555-4726		5:15
5:30			Pam Jeffries				5:30
5:45	Taryn Liebl		hair 555-8720		Jacquie Flynn		5:45
6:00	perm 555-2878		color		tips 555-8047		6:00
6:15					wraps		6:15

the more standard abbreviations are recorded here. The most important thing is that everyone in your salon should know the meaning of the code you are using.

Service	Abbreviation
Shampoo and style	SS
Haircut	HC or X
Permanent wave	Perm
Electrolysis	Elec
Conditioning	C
Hair color	HCL
Body services	BS
Skin care	SC
Lightening	LTN

A client's phone number should be taken in case the requested operator becomes ill or can't make it to work for some reason. Over the time column or next to the name should be a "T" or "R," which will tell if the client is a transit or a request customer. Transit customers are often exchanged in a salon, while request clients cannot be taken from someone's book without the consent of the client.

When the client enters the salon, a diagonal line is drawn through her name, indicating she is in the salon. When she leaves, an "X" is made to indicate that she has left the salon and has paid her bill (by charging or paying cash).

CHAPTER ELEVEN SUMMARY

- The forms you use will determine whether you have on hand the information you will need to run your business.
- The most important record kept in the salon is the appointment book. This should contain information about your clients, how often they come in, and what services they use.

REVIEW QUESTIONS

1. What does the Operator's Monthly Report Sheet show?
2. What must an employee do about reporting tips?
3. What is the single most important record kept in the salon?

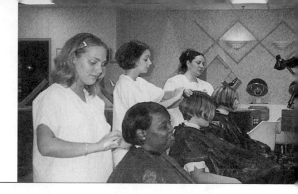

CHAPTER TWELVE

Use of Beauty Schools by Beauty Salons

Many salon owners and managers, as well as operators, overlook one of the most important factors in their careers: keeping up to date. Clients can and do change salons and operators. They feel that their operator or hairstylist is in a rut because he or she does the same hairstyle year after year. Ladies' clothing fashions change each spring and fall; hairstyles, most notably women's, should change at the same time. Unfortunately, by the time the *new look* in hair has been adopted by most salons, the clothing styles have changed several times.

One of the excuses voiced by most operators is that "Mrs. Jones cannot wear the new styles." Sometimes this is true. For the most part, however, clients are looking for a hairstyle that is different, becoming, and up to date. Alert operators and managers make an effort to adapt modern trend styling to suitable styles.

To keep up to date, an operator must practice the new techniques of hairstyling and haircutting. Unfortunately, most operators do not have time during the course of a busy day to experiment with untried and unproven hairstyles. Good beauty schools, on the other hand, have the time to experiment with new styling techniques. Trained instructors stand ready to assist the willing operator or manager with styling in the latest trends. These instructors make a business of producing hairstyles in keeping with the trends desired by most women. Postgraduate styling courses are quite reasonable and, in most cases, tax deductible.

A five-day refresher course each year is recommended to keep your salon and its operators in tune with the times. These five days can be split, with styling shows

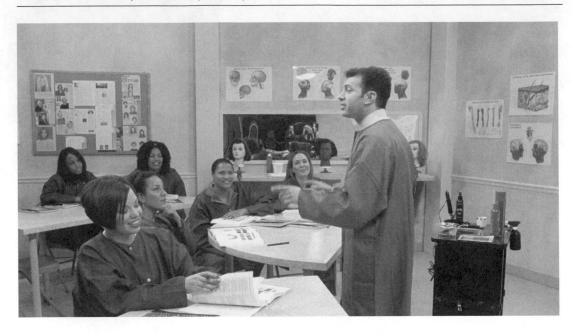

for two days in the spring and the remainder in styling classes and other related classes at the state convention in the fall. Licensed beauty schools do offer one advantage: a chance to practice and experiment under supervision on mannequins and human models. Besides hairstyling classes, beauty schools offer classes in permanent waving, tinting, and salon management.

Specialized Study

Specialized study in permanent hair coloring is offered by several companies manufacturing hair-coloring products. These courses usually run from one to three weeks in length. They are generally held where the main manufacturing plant is located. Such courses consist of a cosmetic science and hair analysis session followed by a practical application session. The color is furnished by the color house giving the classes. The fee is usually quite low, and the courses are often taught through a good beauty school.

Classes in permanent waving are also offered by manufacturers. Like the color classes, these classes are sometimes offered through beauty schools. These classes are usually held on weekends or at night to keep operators from cutting into their day's work.

Some schools offer special courses in electrolysis. This is a special field related to the cosmetic industry. This service, when properly promoted, can produce substantial income for the salon. Operators in this branch of cosmetology are highly paid and respected. More and more managers are finding that they can offer all standard services and still have time for electrolysis treatments. When the electrolysis business has built to the extent that a full-time electrolysis operator is needed, the salon can hire one, thereby giving a new, full-time service to salon customers. Manager-electrologists, who are not directly involved in hairstyling, find that employees no longer look upon them as competitors.

Employment Services

Each year thousands of salons across the country are looking for good, qualified operators to fill vacancies created by operators who have left the industry for some reason. Many of these vacancies result from operators getting married, having children, or moving to another area. Your salon must be ever alert for new talent to replace operators who leave.

Cosmetology schools furnish a service in this area. Each year schools turn out operators of every type to fit the needs of any salon. Schools often keep up-to-date records of students. These records tell where the student (now an operator) is working, what special skills the operator may have acquired since leaving school (such as corrective color, electrolysis, teaching, etc.), and how the operator can be reached. When you need a new employee, first call the local beauty school and state your needs. Most schools are happy to assist in helping an employer obtain the right operator.

In some cases, the school can furnish much needed information regarding a future employee.

Example:

You've run an ad for a new employee. Ten operators have made applications, four were interviewed, and two are selected as possible operators. Ask them which school they attended. A call to the beauty school will aid in making your selection. The school is ready to give information about personality, operator-customer relations, cooperation, attitude, styling ability, promptness, willingness, telephone approach, and cooperation with other operators. After checking on the applicants with the schools, you can make a much better choice of operators.

A special officer at the school usually handles student placement and keeps records on graduates. Usually the school director or the director of personnel, this officer's main job is to help operators and employers get together.

Information Centers

At one time or another, all operators and salon owners have problems. They can be managerial or technical. In either case, a good school with a well-trained, up-to-date staff can help solve some of them or can provide information about where the answer may be found. Here are two examples:

1. During the course of a workday, a woman comes into the salon with a hair-coloring problem. She has tried to color her own hair, and it has turned green. The operator has an idea about how to handle the problem and proceeds. The result of the corrective treatment is not totally perfect. A telephone call to a color expert teaching at a local beauty school might have resulted in the corrective treatment being a complete success. In most cases, trained operators with good working experiences can do a great job; in the case just stated, a conversation with a color instructor could have brought out facts that were not obvious. The result: a perfect corrective job.

2. A salon owner wishes to relocate his salon. The salon owner has his eye on a location but does not know how much business is in that area. From what he can see, it should be a good area. A telephone call to the beauty school placement official will tell him if the other salons in the area are hiring personnel (a good sign) and the approximate business done in that area. The information is obtained by the schools through former students who work in the area and by phone calls from salons in the area requesting staff.

Other information often obtainable from beauty schools includes:

product information (color, permanent waves, relaxers, shampoos, hair spray, setting lotions, etc.)
price schedules for an area
types of salons in the area
styling trends
management procedures

The officer who usually handles this type of information is the school owner or director. If you need technical information, the instructors specializing in the various subjects will be most helpful.

Your ability to work with schools will depend upon the degree of mutual respect that has built up between salons and schools in your community.

CHAPTER TWELVE SUMMARY

- Keeping up to date and adapting modern trends to suitable styles for your clients will keep your clients from looking for new stylists.
- Cosmetology schools may offer specialized studies in hair coloring, permanent waving, or electrolysis.
- Cosmetology schools keep detailed records on students and help salons who need to hire new operators find the right person.
- A good cosmetology school has a well-trained, up-to-date staff that can help solve a wide range of problems encountered by salons in the area.

REVIEW QUESTIONS

1. How many days a year should an operator spend in taking refresher courses?
2. What officer at a cosmetology school usually handles student placement?
3. What information could you get from a beauty school if you were thinking of a particular location for a salon?

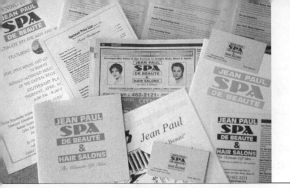

CHAPTER THIRTEEN

Salon Advertising

Before setting up any type of advertising program, be sure to consult with your local state board of cosmetology. Some state boards have definite guidelines that must be followed. Here are two regulations that sometimes appear:

- *All advertising shall state clearly the service being offered and the prices being charged for the said services, and said price or prices as advertised shall not be less than the minimum price adopted in the Judicial District in which the beauty services are offered.*
- *It shall be unlawful and shall be deemed a violation of the minimum price law of the State of _____ for any salon owner, operator, cosmetologist, school, or salon to offer merchandise or other gift premiums or "give-aways" in connection with any beauty service or combination of beauty services unless the total price equals the minimum price of such service or combination of services plus the list or wholesale cost of the merchandise or premium.*

Newspaper Ads

What should be included in a newspaper ad? A newspaper ad should tell a complete story in a short, clear manner. It should have the following features:

1. It should be positioned for the intended reader:
   a. This is done by placing it on a page that is read by potential clients. Some of these pages are social, theater, arts, family living, and radio and

TV. If your salon is connected with a department store, a store page ad will do wonders.

b. Make your ad an eye-catcher. A picture of a good hairstyle, either a drawing or a photograph, will help. An ad with no illustrations will be lost. If you are working on a small budget, place your un-illustrated ad in the personal column.

c. Personalize your ad: "Is your hair. . . ?" "Give yourself . . ." "Do you like. . . ?" "What does this lady?" "for women/men only . . ."; these are a few of the phrases that will help to make your ad more personal. When you make an ad personal, you will attract many more readers than you would if the ad is stated in general terms. Words like *you, your, for women/men only*, etc., will attract the attention you desire.

2. Your ad should state a service or a product:

a. If you wish to advertise a service, try a picture of a hairstyle with the caption "For a more beautiful you" or "For a new hairstyle direct from New York."

b. If you merely wish to advertise a product, try a picture of the product in relation to the hairstyle, or just the hairstyle. A good sentence will help: "Put *color* into your hair" or "Put *curls and bounce* into your hair."

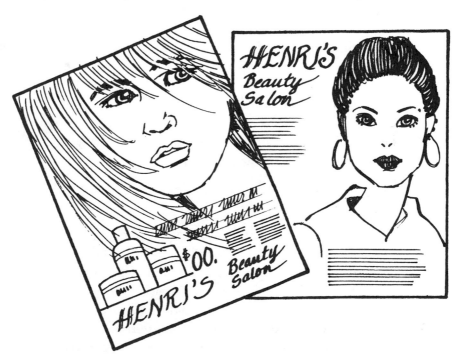

3. Your ad should state a price. This can be a flat price, or it can be an open-ended price stated as a particular amount and up. When stating an open-ended price, be sure that a reason is given for the range: "$??.00 and up, depending upon hair condition and type."

4. All ads should state the normal working hours of the salon. If the salon is open in the evening on some days, this should also be stated.

5. It should state the name of the salon. This should be done in bold, large type if possible.

6. It should state the telephone number of the salon (in large, bold numbers).

7. It should state the location of the salon.

8. It should state the days that the sale will run, when the ad announces a sale.

9. It should be placed on the upper right-hand quarter of odd-numbered pages. Odd-numbered pages are always right-hand pages. When this is impossible, the lower right-hand side of the odd pages is the next choice. If you place an ad on an even-numbered (left-hand) page, be sure that it is at the top corner of the page. The lower left side of the even-numbered pages is next in preference.

10. Run your ad for three days in a row. It will have a greater impact than an ad that is run just once.

11. If you have a unisex salon, be sure to show a picture of both a man and woman in your ad.

12. Since services offered to male customers may be new to them, state clearly what services are available, for example, permanent waving, coloring, etc.

Record Keeping

Be sure to keep a record of all the ads that you have run in the newspaper, and make a booklet of them. On the page that carries the ad, make the following notations:

1. How many calls came in from the ad? This record should be kept by the receptionist for three days after the ad has been run.

2. You should keep a record of all the transient customers who responded and what services were rendered, and note whether they returned for two, three, or more visits. A figure showing the volume of business for the previous year is most helpful in making comparisons.

3. The weather conditions occurring during the time the ad was run should be noted, as it will affect the number of responses. Bad weather discourages

clients. Also, note if there are any major events going on in town at that time. Elections, town celebrations, visiting celebrities, etc., can all affect business volume and response.

Be sure to keep a scrapbook on the advertising done by other salons in your area. A good ad run by a neighboring salon might help you. It can provide a few ideas for future ads of your own.

How to Place an Ad

Ad space can be secured from the newspaper in several ways. The most popular way for a salon using a large amount of newspaper advertising is to purchase it monthly or yearly at special rates. Your entire program of advertising is then planned for a longer period of time and will be arranged to give the salon the best results. Newspapers have artists available who will work with salon managers to plan a program. If you are planning to do a small amount of advertising, then the "each time" method would be the best. This means that you purchase only the space you need for a day or a three-day period. The space is sold in inches or lines of advertising. You pay only for the ad as it is run.

When a salon is open on Monday, Sunday is the best day to advertise in the newspapers. Thursday is the next best day. The other days of the week are equally good, with the exception of Saturday. Saturday is the worst day to advertise for a beauty salon. This is because salons are closed on Sunday, and no phone appointments can be made until Monday morning. By that time the ad is old.

Direct Mail

Because most of a salon's clients usually come from an area surrounding the salon—a five-mile radius is typically where 90 percent of most salons' clients live or work—direct mail makes a lot of sense. Card decks delivered to local homes can be very inexpensive compared to newspapers, and the ad has greater visibility in a card deck because people go through these one at a time. A newspaper may have a circulation of 100,000, but how many of those readers live or work close enough to actually be your clients?

Also, direct mail is the best way to both entice first-time visitors to return to your salon and keep your present clients informed and interested in your services, products, and promotions. A bimonthly newsletter or advertisement promoting your services is an excellent way to stay in touch, and greetings for birthdays and holidays, along with a personal message for other times such as a promotion or a death in the family, are perfect ways to show that you care about your clients.

Word-of-Mouth Advertising

Word-of-mouth advertising is the most effective advertising as well as the least expensive. It is done by clients of beauty salons every day. What makes for good word-of-mouth advertising? First, you must stimulate your clients to talk about your salon in a favorable way. This is achieved by your conversations with them when they are in your salon. When Mrs. Jones visits, be sure to give her all of your time. Find out all her likes and dislikes. Be sure she is happy with your services. Second, be sure that Mrs. Jones always looks her best when she leaves your salon. If you know that she is going to a social affair during the week, but has her hair done on weekends, offer to do a comb-out for her before the affair. This will make her feel good, and she will always return to your salon. Third, if the name of another client comes up, be sure that only the nicest things are said about her. The client in the chair will automatically assume that you say the same about her.

Here are three hints to keep in mind when you are seeking this type of advertising:

1. Always keep your clients looking their best.
2. When working on a client, give him or her your complete attention. Avoid talking to other operators or clients too often.
3. Operators should give clients helpful hints on how to maintain a hairstyle. This should be some simple, workable advice that they can pass on to their friends.

Clubs and Organizations

When you're offered a chance to join a club or organization, do so. You may not want to be an officer of the organization, but the exposure to other members will stimulate business. If employees have a chance to join an organization, encourage them to do so. In fact, if you have to pay their dues, do so. Each time you or a member of your salon staff is seen socially, the topic of hair and beauty salons is bound to come up. In each case, it is a chance to advertise your salon. The more your salon personnel become involved with the community, the better your salon's profits will be.

Always carry plenty of business cards. Hand them out to everybody you meet, and be proud of what you do. "Talk up" your salon and its services at every opportunity; pride and excitement are contagious.

Welcome Wagons and Newcomers' Clubs

Some communities have organizations such as the Welcome Wagon and Newcomers' Club. These organizations call upon new community members and welcome them to the area. They give the newcomer gift items and list the merchants who wish to say "hello." A free gift such as a pen (with your salon name on it) will give you a lot of advertising. Some salons give newcomers special rates on services for their first visit. All these things advertise the salon and generate word-of-mouth advertising.

Sales and Specials

Sales and specials have been used for years, and their attraction has to do with special, low prices or gifts. These sales promotions are still drawing people into salons. Salons use this form of advertising to do two things: stimulate sales and remove old merchandise from the shelves.

Holding too many sales is not good for a salon, as the salon can get the reputation of being a cut-rate operation.

The best time for a sale is when business is at a low during the year; during the peak season it could be a disaster. A special price on children's haircuts will be most effective in late August and early September when children are getting ready to go back to school.

Promotions should follow a specific cycle. Six to eight weeks is a good length for a promotion. The expiration date encourages people to try it before it runs out.

Your salon should always have some type of sale or promotion going, but these should be part of a planned campaign designed to build business where you need it the most: for a new operator, a new service, to bring in more clients, to spark interest in your retail lines, or to enhance your visibility.

Display and Window Advertising

It should be emphasized that, regardless of how good a display may be, it should be changed every three weeks. Displays left longer than that will become dull and lose their effectiveness. If they are changed more often, it will cost too much money, time, and effort. Keep them well lit and colorful, and your clients will enjoy seeing them.

Silent Advertising

Silent advertising can be broken into five different types. All are effective and easy to use.

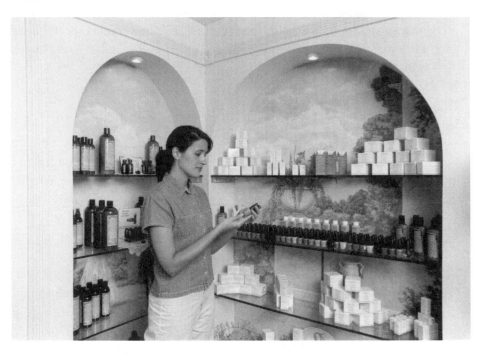

1. *Operators' hairstyles:* The hairstyles of your operators should be done once a week and should be professionally combed when needed. The first impression of what type of styling is done by your salon is from styles shown on your operators. Uncombed hair held by clips or boring styles produce a bad impression. If possible, have all your female operators wear some type of

hair color. In this way, an operator can give clients firsthand information on what hair coloring can do. This is the most effective silent advertising your salon can promote.

2. *Pictures in the styling area are a must:* These should be changed at least once a month. Color pictures will draw more attention than black and white. When using pictures, place two or three large ones in the salon. Small ones, while showing several styles, are usually too small to be effective. When possible, change the background of the pictures once a month. For example, in January have a picture with a black background or border and a gold frame. In February have a picture with a red background or border and a gold frame, and so on.

3. *Magazine articles:* An article in a magazine (on display in the salon), written by a beauty specialist, beauty consultant, salon owner, or manager, can help sell all kinds of items from conditioners to face powders. You could print your own newsletter under a title such as "If You Ask Me." Your replies to beauty questions will become your sales message. The nice thing about this type of advertising is that the person is already sold before the sale attempt has started.

4. *Styling aids and cosmetic items:* Styling aids and cosmetics used on a client's hair are easy to sell because the client has seen the operator use the product professionally and likes the idea of having her own professional product. Everything that the operator uses at the station to set and style the client's hair should be retailed. Your best advertising displays for this type of merchandise are a clean, neat working cabinet for your operators and a well-stocked, well-lit, immaculately clean display rack in the reception area.

5. *Pens, appointment cards, key tags, business-card magnets, etc.:* These inexpensive giveaway items (with salon advertising on them) are another means of silent advertising. They can be purchased in volume and stored, since they will not spoil. It's amazing how a pen will pass from one person to another in the course of a couple of days.

Style Shows and Demonstrations

Style shows and demonstrations are a great form of advertising for a beauty salon because you have the attention of an interested, captive audience. The people you are demonstrating to are interested in what you have to say and will listen. Each hairstyle you create during a demonstration should be explained, and the care of it should be discussed. Related subjects, such as tinting, bleaching, or permanent waving, can all be introduced while you are working on the model.

Fashion shows can be a great form of advertising. Most salons miss taking best advantage of advertising because they are unsure of how to go about it. Normally, a clothing store will approach a salon for help on a fashion show. The salon styles the models' hair and re-combs the hair after each costume change. Unfortunately, usually the only credit given to the salon is a two-line recognition ad on a program that everyone leaves on the table or throws into the trash immediately after the show.

To get maximum effect from this form of advertising, someone must explain the hairstyles on the models. Most mistresses of ceremonies will welcome the aid of a beauty salon manager or owner in presenting and narrating the program. Be sure that the hairstyle or color service of each operator is noted and that full credit is given.

Business Lunches

Business lunches or morning breakfasts of such groups as the Chamber of Commerce, the Lions Club, Junior League, and Rotary are good avenues to male clients. Salons can coordinate hairstyles on men with styles from a good men's store. A lecture class on hair and nail care is also good advertising. Be sure to have a number of before-and-after pictures available for viewing.

Public Relations

It was once said that a good public relations man was a fellow who could pay for a cup of coffee and get a client to sign a million dollar contract. For many years, salon public relations work fell only on the shoulders of the owner or manager. This is not true today. Each operator must do a certain amount of public relations work if he or she wants to make a good living and ensure the success of the salon. There are several ways you can promote good public relations. Here are five:

1. *The manager speaks to each customer entering the salon:* If the manager does not know the person's name, he or she can wait until the person is seated at

an operator's chair and take the name from the appointment book. Everyone likes to be noticed. The greatest recognition is the one in which you mention a person's name. "Hello, Mrs./Mr. Jones; it sure is a nice day today." This type of greeting will keep customers in the salon year after year.

2. *The salon manager keeps active in the community:* Volunteer to provide the elderly with a free shampoo and set one day a year. If you do this, you can get the newspaper to carry an article in the local paper at no cost to you. The friends and relatives of these people will hear about their kind treatment, and good will is firmly established. Also, help out on fund-raising events by making the salon a drop-off point for clothing collections, etc.

3. *Operator-client relations must be on a personal level:* This can be as simple as taking a client's coat, brushing his or her suit off after a hair shaping, or saying "Happy Birthday." To do this well, each operator must have a file on each of her steady customers. When something important happens, it should be noted and mentioned to the client the next time she comes into the salon.

Example:

Mrs. Jones was elected president of her bridge club. The notice came out on Tuesday. On Friday when she comes in for her appointment, her operator would say, "Congratulations, I see you were elected president of your bridge club. I sure am happy you were elected."

With this kind of relationship, the salon down the street will be unlikely to take Mrs. Jones away from her present operator.

4. *Use the mail:* When an operator finds that one of her clients is sick, in the hospital, or has a death in the family, she should inform the salon manager. A card should be sent to the client, signed by the salon manager and the operator. Always send holiday and birthday greetings. The small cost of this is a good investment in a client who may spend several hundred dollars a year in your salon and bring more clients in to sample your services and products.

5. *Take bad P.R. out of complaints:* One of the most difficult things to handle in the salon is the complaint. The client is usually upset, and, the more she talks about her trouble, the more emotional she becomes. The first thing to do is to talk softly and find out what the problem is. Next, admit nothing until you have spoken to your operator, but try to find out what the client wants to have done. In the case of unsatisfactory work, try to have her

return to the salon to have the problem corrected. If an adjustment is in order, make it as quickly and quietly as possible. She may not like what she has experienced, but, if the situation is handled carefully, she will not damn you to all her neighbors.

Advertising through Conventions and Educational Seminars

Conventions and seminars are a real learning experience. When an operator returns, he or she will have some new ideas, some new styles, and some new ambitions. The salon should capitalize on this. When the operator or manager returns, an ad should be run to inform clients.

Example:

"Mr. John has returned from New York, where he has been attending a hair-styling seminar. He has brought back with him many new hairstyles suited to the new fall clothing."

The added business from such an ad sometimes pays for the trip. The main thing to remember is that, if you are going to do something, let someone know about.

Salon Conversation—A Form of Advertising

If operators are not talking to one another in the salon, you are missing one of the best forms of advertising. The talking should not be going on all the time, nor should it distract from the client, but it is a very good form of advertising. During the course of the day you might ask a nearby operator, "Jan, how do you like your new hair coloring?" This is like a spot advertising notice in the store. Immediately, all eyes in the salon will turn to Jan. As Jan says she likes it, all the operators and clients will automatically start talking about hair coloring. This type of advertising is quite effective and is a good way to break up a day's work. If it is done too often, however, it will lose its effectiveness.

Several other advertising plans are used each day by salons throughout the country. Not all of the ones presented here are equally effective in all salons. The main thing is to try them and see how they work.

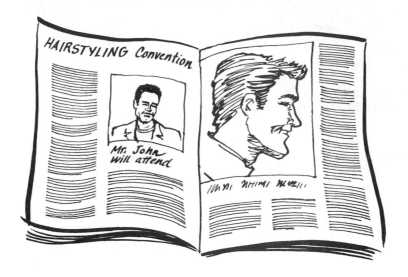

CHAPTER THIRTEEN SUMMARY

- Some state boards have adopted regulations that must be followed in any advertising program.
- A newspaper ad should tell a complete story in a short, complete manner.
- Direct mail can target potential customers in the area around your salon.
- Word-of-mouth advertising is the most effective and the cheapest type of advertising.
- The more exposure you and your operators have in the community, the more your business will become known and will grow.

REVIEW QUESTIONS

1. How long should a newspaper ad be run?
2. What is the most important fact to record about a newspaper ad?
3. What is the most effective type of advertising?
4. When is the best time to run a sale?
5. Who in a salon is responsible for public relations?

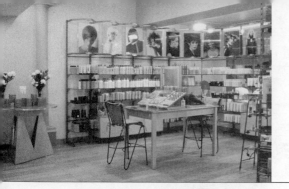

CHAPTER FOURTEEN

Merchandising (Selling) in a Beauty Salon

One of the questions most asked among salon owners when they get together is "How are sales?" or "How's business?" The answers to these questions are as confusing as the questions themselves. The normal reply is "Things are going fine" or "We're ahead of last year." From these questions and answers it's obvious that many salon owners fail to comprehend the full meaning of the salon business. One manager might think of business in terms of customer service while another may consider the overall operation of the salon.

To keep that from happening in this chapter, a few terms should be defined:

Merchandising in the beauty salon is the total of activities related to selling all goods, services, and retail items that one might find in a beauty salon.

Gross sales is the total amount of money taken in by the salon during the year.

Net profit is the difference between the cost of goods and services and their selling price. Labor would be part of the cost of a shampoo and set service as well as the shampoo, wave set, and hair spray.

Real profit is a term used to describe the amount of money left after all bills have been paid.

Main Steps in Merchandising

With these terms in mind, let us explore how to merchandise in a beauty salon. This chapter centers around three main steps and how to use them. If these steps are followed, the salon will prosper and grow.

1. Get customers into the salon.
2. Give customers what they want.
3. Sell customers what they need.

Get Customers into the Salon

What makes a customer come into a salon? Some of the frequently heard answers to this question are location, salon appearance, a telephone listing and display ad, and good recommendations. All of these and many more are very important to all salon owners. But, in addition, a salon must launch and maintain an active program to get customers into the salon and retain them as customers. You are now talking about spending money, and in business you don't gamble with money. You invest it wisely in sound, firm, tried, and tested approaches to making more money. Presented here are a few items that work. However, keep your eyes and mind open for new ideas that appear to fit your operation.

Planning. First make a plan, then follow it. In setting up the plan consider the following questions.

1. What type of customers are you looking for?
2. What type of customers come into your salon?
3. Do you wish to change the type of customers you already have, or do you wish to just add a few more?
4. Should you consider changing your location? (You will not serve too many movie stars in Smalltown, U.S.A.!)
5. What types of businesses are near your salon, and what is their traffic pattern?
6. Can you tie in with their advertising program for the benefit of your salon?

Take the time, answer all these questions, and write them on a piece of paper.

Example:

The name of our salon is the Shady Lakes Beauty Salon, located in the Shady Lakes Shopping Center. The customers are mostly residents in the area with some customers from other parts of town. The customers are middle-income housewives and white-collar workers with an average of two years of college. Families have about two children each between the ages of four and eighteen.

The objective is to increase the number of customers while keeping the present ones.

We will want our salon as close to the major pedestrian traffic centers in the shopping area as possible. This will be next to the drug store, dress shop, barber shop, cosmetic store, department store, or supermarket.

Next we will want to contact the shops next to us and see what they are doing in relation to promotion. Each month, merchants have a gimmick to draw customers. Let the merchants who do a lot of advertising set the theme of the promotions and sales. If the dress store has a pre-spring sale, and it is located next door to our salon, we will take advantage of it. Decorate our window to read "Swing into Spring with a New Hairstyle." Use colors that will blend but not be overpowered by our neighbor's display.

Since this is a shopping center (with a regular group of customers), chances are that people are used to shopping in the same stores. Our window display will attract some, yet others may not see it, so a reinforcement is needed. Since this is a dress sale, have the clerks in the dress store come in for a new spring hairdo. When Mrs. Jones goes in to purchase a new dress, she sees Marge's hair and comments upon it. This is good for two reasons; first, Marge is flattered, and second, the customer is told where she got her new hairstyle. The cost of this type of advertising is very little, and the results pay off.

Salon Appearance. The overall appearance of a salon is a real asset to your business. Attractive windows and doors have already been discussed, but they are so important to business that they are worth mentioning again. Clean windows with attractive displays, changed every three weeks, are real business builders.

Be sure that the waiting area is well lighted and open so passersby can see into the salon at night. The cost is low, and benefits, both for advertising and protection, are large.

Welcome Wagon. Have your operators help advertise your salon by offering discount prices through "Welcome Wagon" services, where new people are greeted by the community. The discount is usually offered to the new client on her first visit to a salon. This will bring new clients in, but be sure that the difference between the discount price and the normal price is credited to the operator's pay.

You can defeat the whole purpose if sloppy work is done because it is offered at a discount.

As an alternative to a discount, you can offer a free retail gift with haircut, color, or perm. The client will receive a good value, it will cost you far less than the value to the client, and you will have introduced one of your high-profit retail items to a potential buyer.

Meetings and Training Seminars. Hold shop meetings at least once a month during off hours and have a guest stylist or teacher present the program. These meetings should last about three hours, and attendance must be mandatory for all operators. Once operators learn that the meetings are worthwhile, they will attend voluntarily. Be sure these programs are well planned and interesting.

Some of the things that should be stressed during these meetings are human relations, telephone techniques, salesmanship, new hairstyles, new products, and techniques. Give your operators training in how to meet people and what to talk about.

Since you have made some effort to get clients into the salon, help your operators with ideas on how to keep them. Manufacturers, distributors, and salon educators offer this instruction; seek them out and let them help you. One important thing to remember is that, while you might own the salon, the operators own the business. If you don't believe it, visualize losing your entire crew.

Electronic Media. Many fine training videotapes and audiocassettes, spanning every subject from cuts and hair color to client service, are available from salon education companies. The tapes can train and can stimulate lively discussions. You can also construct your own program using the materials mentioned.

High School Demonstrations. Demonstrations at high schools are always welcome and represent a source of future customers. The one thing you must know, however, is what audience you are going to do a show for and what their ages are. Speaking of ages, if teenagers are wearing their hair in a style popular among peers, don't try to change it. Don't insist on any particular length. It is better to have teens come in for a trim once a month than not at all. When speaking to teenage groups who wear their hair natural, stress cleanliness (shampoo that you sell), hair trims (as a cure for split ends), and facial cleansers and makeup (cosmetics that you sell). Don't talk about things that will offend and drive these new customers from your door.

If the group is older, talk about permanent waves and hair coloring. Always bring items your salon sells, and don't discuss items that can be purchased elsewhere.

The Telephone Book. The telephone book is a source of advertising if used properly. Yellow page ads should be large enough to be seen but should not be overpowering. The name of the salon, the location, and the phone number must be included.

Operators' names are sometimes placed in ads and do wonders for holding operators in your salon. Shears, combs, and hairstyles are sometimes illustrated, and do dress up an ad. These take up space, however, and space is money, so use it wisely.

If the salon has evening hours, they should be stated in the ad. Products and brand names have been used in ads, but, when these products can be found in any well-stocked drug store and easily purchased, they are not as effective. Be sure to stock and advertise only those products sold exclusively through salons.

Credit cards that the salon will accept should be mentioned in the ad since this has proven to be a real drawing card.

Word-of-Mouth. Nothing but good can come to a salon that has its clients working for it. Word-of-mouth is the best type of advertising. Doctors, dentists, and attorneys have relied on this type of advertising for years. If your salon has a customer who has sent you a client, be sure to send her a thank-you note. A new and steady client can mean hundreds of dollars a year to a salon, and this type of lead *deserves* a "thank you."

This type of courtesy can be acknowledged by a card, a short note, or a small gift when the helpful client comes in the next time. In thanking a person, be sure to mention the name of the new customer:

"Mrs. Jones, I want to thank you for recommending this salon to Mrs. Roberts." You might even add, "Please accept this gift as a token of our appreciation."

These techniques for getting the customer into the salon have, no doubt, brought other ideas to your mind. At this point, write them down in your notebook and form a plan of action.

"Bring-a-friend" promotions often produce excellent results. Offer a free discount or free products to new clients and to your present clients who referred them.

Note: The happier your present clients are with your service, the better this promotion works.

Give Customers What They Want

When clients come into the salon, they are looking for two things—service and satisfaction. Give the client what he or she wants. Upon arrival, greet the person immediately, especially if it is a client's first visit. Should the person have to wait, offer a magazine or a cup of coffee to help pass the waiting time.

When the person is finally placed in the styling chair, be sure to listen to what the client wants. (Admittedly, a few customers ask the impossible, and, if this is the case, some compromise must be reached.) Don't try to sell a client everything in the salon on the first visit. The first visit should be the time for the client to get to know the salon and the operators. The first and main objective of this visit is to gain the person's confidence and to get to know one another.

Ask the Right Questions. Ask questions that can add to sales promotion later on. Some of these questions are:

Are you going anywhere special?
What have you been doing interesting lately?
What does your husband/wife do for a living?
How many children do you have?
Do you work?
What do you expect from this style?
Do you play (bridge, tennis, golf, etc., whichever fits the person)?
Do you belong to any organizations?
What is your birthday?

Not all these questions are asked of all customers all the time. You might ask only one or two of them on the first visit. You might get her started, and she will fill you in on the rest without your asking.

Here is a typical conversation and how a smart stylist will use the information:

Operator: *Mrs. Jones, how did you hear about us?*
Customer: Mrs. Smith recommended you to me.
Operator: *She is a nice person. Do you play bridge with her?*
Customer: Yes, our husbands work together and we have a lot of the same friends.
Operator: *Now that we have your hair shampooed, how would you like it cut and styled?*
Customer: Something special; I have a party to go to tonight.
Operator: *That sounds great. Do you have any children?*
Customer: Yes, I have two, Jim is seven, and Cathy is thirteen.
Operator: *I bet you keep pretty busy. Do you work, too?*
Customer: Yes, I work at the Jones Corporation up the street.

From this short conversation the smart stylist has learned several important things about this customer. She should write them on her client record card and use them for sales information later. Some of the information she has received is:

1. She is employed by the X manufacturing firm, and her husband must be making about the same amount as Mrs. Smith's husband. (Useful in determining taste and income.)
2. She has two children, and the girl is a potential customer.
3. The daughter can use shampoo, hair conditioner, and styling aids.
4. She can come in for an appointment after work or very early in the morning.
5. She will be a potential advertising customer since she comes in contact with many people in her work.
6. Due to an active life and her work, she will want a style that is conservative and easy to care for but which can be adapted from time to time for special occasions.
7. Don't make her look like a carbon copy of Mrs. Smith, who will no doubt be at the same parties.

Go Slow at the Onset. On the customer's initial visit, the operator should be polite and courteous. Make sure that the customer is pleased before she leaves. It is important that the operator does not use high-pressure sales techniques on the first exposure.

Ask the Client to Return. The most important thing is that the operator invite the client back to the salon. The operator can do this by saying "Can I make an appointment for your next (service)?" Should the client prefer to call in, the operator should give a card to the person with the name of the salon and operator's name on it. If no response is forthcoming in a month, be sure the client receives an operator's check sheet for customer service. This is a nice way to say "We enjoy your business."

Sell Customers What They Need

Selling is no game; it is a business, and, like all businesses, reward (pay) should be given for the effort rendered by the salesperson. Too often a salon stocks retail items only to have them grow dusty on the shelves. If the operator and the receptionist are paid an additional amount to sell these items, the salon will profit.

Pay a 15 percent commission to the person who does the selling. If you pay this with a separate check, at a separate time from regular paychecks, you will focus more attention on the money that can be earned from retail product sales. Also, if you keep a chart of retail performance, noting each operator's performance over time and his or her performance compared with the others' for the month, you have an excellent motivational tool.

Sales and selling take very little extra effort, and the profits will startle you. Here are a few practical examples of how to sell.

Example:

When Mrs. Jones comes in for her next appointment, the conversation can be guided by the operator in a manner that will produce an extra sale or sales. "Mrs. Jones, we have just gotten in some of the best shampoo I have ever used. It thoroughly cleans the scalp and hair and, most important, leaves the hair easy to manage. It's acid balanced so that it will not strip color or harm a permanent wave. It is also good for split hair ends. If you are looking for a shampoo for the whole family, I would certainly recommend it."
or
"Mrs. Jones, I have noticed that your hair spray seems to be building up on your hair shaft. This will eventually make your hair look dull. I'm going to use a new hair spray right now to finish styling your hair. It's water soluble, so it washes out when you shampoo. Why don't you try a bottle and have some fun seeing what you can do with it at home? I'll give you some pointers."

This type of selling will greatly increase salon profits. The operator gets the commission on the first can, and, if the receptionist is sharp, she will sell additional items to the customer.

A good receptionist can also increase the gross income of a salon. When a client calls for an appointment, the receptionist always asks if he or she wants a manicure, lash and brow tint, eyebrow arch, or a conditioner—services that are often overlooked. For this added effort she should be given a percentage of the profits over a certain figure. Usually this is 2 to 5 percent. She should also earn 15 percent on retail sales that she is able to make.

How to Purchase, Advertise, and Sell Retail Items

Generally speaking, all purchasing should be done by one person. The items purchased should fall into two classes, usable items (stock) and retail items (items for sale). Ordering is governed by the "want list" and the inventory sheet. Amounts of such items should fall into a pattern reflecting the traffic flow of the salon. Care should be taken to supply the salon with an adequate stock.

Selecting Retail Lines

The lines you choose will have a lot to do with your success in retail sales. Here are some important points to keep in mind when selecting lines:

1. Don't buy into too many lines. Three, four at the most, are what a salon can move effectively.
2. Be sure the lines are popular with your staff, as operators usually sell most effectively when they understand and like a product.
3. Be sure the lines are sold exclusively to salons. Any diversion (sales to mass marketers) will undermine your sales and your credibility. If you do find one of your lines being sold in local mass markets, contact the distributor and manufacturer. If you don't get satisfaction, drop that line.
4. You are buying into a distributor, not just a line. Go with the distributor who offers you the most promotional help with such offers as shrink wraps, promotions, special deals, education, etc. Build a relationship with this distributor instead of wasting your time saving nickels and dimes on a few products.

Retail Items

Choosing which retail items to sell is by far the most important decision. Before entering this field, ask yourself the following questions:

1. Who are my customers?
2. How much money do they have?
3. What will they purchase?
4. Who is to do the selling?

If the operators and receptionist are going to do the selling, be sure they are paid for it. The customers in most areas require different things at different times. One item or a group of related items should be featured each month or, at the very least, every two months.

Markup

The markup should be high enough to cover the cost of the items and still make a good profit. One word of caution: don't overprice your goods; remember, you have competition down the street at the local drug store and dress shop.

In most cases, the product will be priced at twice the purchase price. This amounts to a 50 percent markup because 50 percent of the product's retail price is markup. While this price may vary, the 50 percent markup is a good rule of thumb for specialty stores such as salons, where professional recommendations are very important and where merchandising does not rely on the high turnover of mass marketing.

The Yearly Promotion

After you have looked at the customers, their incomes, and what their needs might be, you are now ready to set up a yearly sales promotion program. Here is one for your consideration. You must adapt it to your own area, and remember that it takes time to build up a demand for new types of merchandise. Don't suddenly go into selling clothing or jewelry in a big way. You need to make a long-term commitment, and start small, to see if it will work without risking too much of your capital.

January (Hair Spray Sale)
The can should carry the salon name and be used by all your operators at their stations. Say that a can of spray costs the salon $2.00. It should retail for about $4.00. However, during the month of January, offer the can of spray to all your customers at the special price of $2.00. If they like the spray, you will have a customer who will give you a profit of about $1.00 a can all the rest of the year.

Note: The average woman uses a can of spray a month if she is having her hair done at the salon. She will use two cans per month if she has a daughter who also uses hair spray. Why should she purchase this product at the drug store?

February (Shampoo with Cut)
If shampoo sells in your salon for $4.00/8-ounce bottle, you can give your clients a $4.00 value for $2.00 (your cost at 50 percent markup)—less if you get a special deal from your distributor. Offer a free bottle of professionally

prescribed shampoo for each client getting a haircut during the month of February. You must have several types of the shampoo on hand—fine, normal, oily, colored/permed hair, for example—so that your operators can prescribe the type best for the client. This not only builds up demand for your shampoo but it builds up your operators' reputation as experts.

March (Wind Bonnets, Rain Hats, and Umbrellas)

A variety of these, well displayed, can sell fast. You might have your operators or receptionist wear them as a promotional idea. These items should be low cost. If you sell umbrellas, keep them under $10.00. The $10.00 figure seems to have some magic about it when selling in a beauty salon.

April (Swing into Spring with a New Hairdo)

Promote permanent waving and hair coloring. Retail items such as hair bows, fancy combs, false curls, and the like should all be promoted. If you are going to sell them effectively, see that your operators wear the items themselves. Your operators and receptionist are your prime advertising media. Permanent wave cards, sent to customers for special discounts during this month, are a good idea as well.

May (A Gift for Mother)

Gift certificates for beauty service should be actively promoted to each client known to have a living mother. Here is a place where a good reception room display can help. Again, have operators participate as much as possible.

May–June (Graduation)

Gifts for the high school and college students should be stressed at this time. Styling tools of all kinds, fancy brushes, combs, and the like are good retail items. Be sure to have several gift boxes available, and have these items well displayed.

June–July–August (Skin Care)

Suntan lotion, skin conditioners, skin shield, cleansing creams, etc., all should be promoted during the summer months as a safeguard against the harmful effects of the sun. A promotion of "Try our new makeup" is good. Beach hats, sunglasses, swimming caps, small cans of hair spray, combs, and brushes are all good selling items. Be sure the displays are well taken care of in the reception room.

September–October (Back to School)

Promote haircuts or shaping for children going back to school. Also, you might get a list of all the teachers in your local school system and send them a card for 10 percent off any permanent wave. This is also a good month to talk to girls' clubs such as Blue Birds, Camp Fire Girls, Girl Scouts, etc. Topics can range from hair care to skin care, with special emphasis on correcting dry skin and hair conditions resulting from summer activities, that is, too much sun, chlorine in swimming pools, etc.

November (Football Season)

Knit gloves, scarves, and hats are good sellers this month. Hair conditioners, brushes, and combs should also be good sellers.

December (Christmas, Hanukkah, Kwanza)

Gifts of all kinds that can be used as "stocking stuffers" go well; gift certificates and small items are well worth stocking at this time of year. This is also the season to empty the shelf of all the merchandise you don't want or use. If you are going to have a sale, now is the time. Your receptionist can gift wrap the items at no extra charge if purchases are made before the client's appointment. What better way to have her wait on those December days! Items for men should be stocked during this month and should include after-shave lotion, colognes, combs, and brushes.

Advertising Retail Items

You have probably noticed that most of the promotion of services and retail items is done on a personal basis in the salon. Newspaper ads, while good, are no substitute for personal selling. The more personal an approach, such as cards through the mail, a telephone call, or direct talking to a group, the better.

Percent Markup

After you decide on a year's program and the products you wish to sell, the next problem is "How much do I mark up the item?" In most cases, the markup is about 50 percent. Be sure that you keep in mind that you are in competition with the local drug and department stores down the street. Another good rule is to sell only items that are exclusively yours in the impulse buy area.

When it is time for a special sale, make sure obvious savings are involved. Reduce all sale items to an extremely low figure.

Example:

A $2.00 item for $.50. This will not only clean the shelves but produce a lot of good will. Do not place anything on sale that you have sold at full price recently.

Cosmetics

The sale of facial cosmetics has certain special problems and risks but is a source of extra salon income. You may want to carry a full line from one cosmetic house or another. Be sure to do this under consignment. Shades and fashions change so fast that you don't want to be left holding the bag with too much unsold stock. If you do decide to retail such items, look for a good supplier. Be sure your staff supports the line and uses it. It helps if your receptionist is also your makeup specialist.

Items such as nail polish can be handled successfully and should be the responsibility of the manicurist in the salon. She has the time for selling hand creams and nail polish. Usually operators are not interested in this type of thing and will not promote it well.

The sale of dresses, blouses, and hose should be done in a separate area. Hair spray that floats in the air can ruin a good dress in a matter of days. (A few salons do combine the areas, but most of the time it does not meet with much success.)

Important Rules

When merchandising in a salon, keep the following in mind:

1. Know your customer.
2. Know what you are selling.
3. Know who is going to sell it.
4. Know how much it costs and what kind of profit you intend to make.

At the end of the year be sure to evaluate what you have sold and the profits made from such sales. Then plan another sales program and carry it through.

CHAPTER FOURTEEN SUMMARY

- The three steps in merchandising are getting the customer into the salon, giving customers what they want, and selling customers what they need.
- A salon must launch and maintain an active program to get new customers in and retain them as customers.

- All purchasing, of usable items and retail items, should be done by one person. Choosing a retail line is a very important decision; a good distributor can help with promotions and education.
- To merchandise in a salon know your customers, know what you are selling, know who will sell it, and know your costs and what kind of profit you will make.

REVIEW QUESTIONS

1. What is real profit?
2. What do Welcome Wagon services do?
3. What commission should be paid for retail sales in a salon?
4. Why should cosmetics be carried only under consignment?

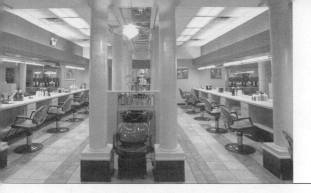

Key Points for Successful Salon Operation Reviewed

A salon that is conceived on paper and developed with wood, textiles, stone, water, and electricity will eventually become a living establishment. Salons, like people, have personalities. The personality is formed in the same way that a person's personality is formed. Personality is dependent upon original composition (actual materials), the brains (management), the working parts or organs (operators), the support systems (supplies and maintenance), and, finally, the work it produces. A salon that is proud, has a good working staff, has adequate support systems, and produces quality workmanship will live a long and prosperous life.

Its owners will profit both by financial and emotional rewards. Like human families, some salons will be good and some will have trouble. The main thing is to establish what causes a salon to do well and then make sure everything is done to put it on the right track. Any salon that is functioning well can be said to have a good personality. A salon's personality is governed by five main components. If any one of these breaks down or is not used, it will suffer. They are:

1. the original composition
2. the management
3. the working staff
4. the support systems
5. the product

All the parts must function well, or the salon will fall into trouble. If the trouble is not corrected, the salon will soon die.

Original Composition

Regardless of how the salon is started, or who owns it, it must be well built. Some of the most important things to check when purchasing a salon or starting a new one are:

1. *Walls, floor, and ceiling.* All of these must be easy to maintain. They must be sturdy and not need constant repair.

    Example:

    A salon whose ceiling is cracked and has plaster coming loose will not speak highly of its owners or managers. The floor should be replaced before it completely wears out and becomes decomposed. The walls should be constantly maintained. Chipped paint, dirty wallpaper, or loose wooden panels all give a salon a bad image.

2. *Plumbing and electrical connections.* These should be checked and maintained at least once a month, and repairs should be made when needed. Plumbing drains and pipes should be cleaned with a good pipe and drain solvent. This solvent should keep the plumbing free from hair and other buildup. Hot and cold water taps should be checked for leaks, and faucet washers should be replaced as needed. Shampoo hoses should be changed when worn out. Electrical outlets and lights should be constantly checked and replaced when needed. Burned-out lights indicate neglect.

3. *Dryers.* These should be cleaned and maintained on a regular basis. If this is done, they will perform well. A dirty dryer or one that has a loose connection can develop a smell as bad as a person who hasn't had a bath in a month.

4. *Brushes, combs, and manicuring equipment.* These must be constantly replaced and always be in perfect condition.

5. *Towels.* These should be replaced as needed and kept extremely clean.

Management

Management, the brains of the salon, must make the decisions and motivate the workforce. Here is a brief summary of what the salon management (owners and managers) must do in order to perform well.

1. *Attend to the needs of all parts of the salon:* From the physical condition of the salon to the nuances of psychology, the responsibility for observing these

and reacting to them falls on the management. They work together as a whole, and thus none can be neglected without detriment to the others.

2. *Help the staff succeed:* By helping each staff person succeed, the management builds a strong, loyal staff. Also, the salon's success depends on the success of each person working in it.

3. *Allow the staff to participate:* Nothing will build up resentment among employees in any business faster than feeling that they have no voice in their own future. Allowing people a voice, at least in an advisory capacity, builds each person's sense of worth, and that is important to good performance and good relationships. Also, employees really do have much that is valuable to contribute. While the management retains control over final decision making, by tapping the various resources among the staff they will find that the whole is truly greater than the sum of its parts.

4. *Develop your own management skills:* Management is not easy, but education makes it less difficult. Invest in management training. You will find many answers there and also others with whom to share your feelings and whom you can call on for an objective voice during difficult times.

Working Staff

From Chapter 8, we see that it takes money and time to select the right employees. Too often employees seem to function well alone but do not, or will not, function with one another. Helping your employees work together is called teamwork. It is your job as a salon owner and manager to coordinate your operators to work as a team in your salon. No good salon has operators working only in pairs, or by themselves. It must be a team effort. The army has a phrase for this: "esprit de corps." Here are a few ways that you can develop salon spirit:

1. *Uniforms and uniform changes:* You would not like eating beans three meals a day for ten years. Your operators feel that way about their uniforms. Uniforms should be changed as the seasons change (color and style) to keep up the morale of the operators. This also helps keep the uniforms in good condition as the same one is not worn constantly, and, of course, the uniforms should be kept in excellent condition at all times.

2. *Operator's thank you:* It is interesting that a new operator is the one that receives the most attention, while the steady, hardworking, durable

employees seem to be forgotten. When a new employee is hired, the employer is willing to spend $3,000.00 or more to get him or her started. This figure includes guaranteed salaries, advertising, and special promotions. After an employee has been with the business for five years, she is actually making money for the salon. Instead of being praised for her efforts and the time she has worked for the firm, she is often taken for granted.

Spend a few dollars occasionally on a gift for your operators to let them know how much you appreciate their work. A dinner party will do the same thing. Honest praise is a valuable management tool; use it.

3. *Help all you can in the salon:* Cooperation is contagious. Helping with a shampoo here or with a few rollers there will get many extra dollars' worth of effort out of your operators. When you are making a decision about the salon, ask the employees to help you; whether you take their advice or not, makes no difference—they still like to be asked.

4. *Find out as much as you can about your employees' personalities:* As much as you can, place each operator next to someone he or she can cooperate with. Never place two experienced operators or two new operators together. This will start a young section and an older section in the salon. Pair young, new stylists with older, more experienced ones. The older ones will teach the new ones new and old methods of doing things. The young operator will keep the older one motivated.

Support Systems

Support systems include your bookkeeping system, supply room, supply system, working capital, receptionist, and maintenance department. Like food, the support system will nourish, feed, and revitalize your salon. It can keep it running in a good, smooth, profitable fashion. Let us look at each of these things separately.

Bookkeeping System

If you were expecting a check on the first of the month and it did not come until the fifteenth, you would not be pleased. Your employees feel the same way about their paychecks. Be sure that the bookkeeper is prompt about paying your help and that the checks are accurate. Nothing is worse than a late check or one that is not correct.

Supply Room and Supplies

This is one area where mistakes can really cost the salon money. Your employees should know what supplies are available to them, which supplies can be ordered, and when supplies are due to run out. When operators go into the supply room, they should be able to find what they want and have it readily available. If they are constantly making substitutions or doing without things, they will soon become discouraged, and their productivity will fall off. This causes hard feelings on both the operator's and manager's parts.

Working Capital

A salon must have enough working capital (in cash and checking account) to make change, cash checks, and pay bills. A receptionist should never have to go out of the salon to look for change. Also, you should have enough money to keep the business in operation for two months without having to worry about closing the salon. Too often a salon has to cut down on hours because there is not enough working capital.

Receptionist

The receptionist is the nerve center of the salon. He or she is the one who will keep the whole system running smoothly. The receptionist's duties should be well defined and known to everyone in the salon. Knowing the job's limits of authority and responsibility, the receptionist will be able to keep everyone happy. The receptionist is the salon's number one public relations officer and must reflect the best image for your salon. A strain on this person can throw the whole system into a downward spin.

Maintenance Department

A salon that is constantly disorderly and dirty will self-destruct. You must hire a good maintenance person. Some of this person's duties should be to clean the windows, doors, and walls and to paint them when needed; he or she should care for the restrooms, change lightbulbs when needed, etc.

The Product

This is the end result. Each client who leaves the salon should look and feel his or her best—look good, feel good, and want to return as soon as possible. If all the factors that are in the salon's personality are functioning well, the salon will succeed. The main thing to consider here is that the final product, whether it is a hairstyle, permanent wave, hair color, or a haircut, should be up to date, look great, and be professionally done. It should look good enough for you to be able to tell a friend "That style came from my salon." When the client is leaving, make sure that someone says, "We have enjoyed serving you; please come back soon."

With a system like this, in which all parts function perfectly, you can't help but have a successful salon.

Checklist for Starting a Salon

The following checklist is designed to help you keep track of the steps necessary to start your own salon.

1. Decide on how to finance your operation.
2. Choose your location and check zoning regulations.
3. Negotiate your lease after you know what improvements will be needed and at what cost.
4. Obtain needed permits, insurance, and access to public utilities.
5. Select your equipment.
6. Design your interior, exterior, and front window display, keeping in mind the clientele you would like to attract.
7. Select magazines, books, and newspapers for the waiting area, again keeping your clientele in mind.
8. Stock and arrange your supply room.
9. Set up pay schedules for the various personnel you will need.
10. Place ads in the classified section of newspapers and magazines to obtain salon personnel.
11. Set grooming and clothing policies.
12. Try to determine the actual expenses of the salon.
13. Keep records of clients, employees, sales, and profits.

14. Decide on how to merchandise your salon.
15. Set up an advertising program.
16. Explore periodic refresher courses for yourself and your staff.

Checklist for an Attractive Decor

Consult an interior decorator in order to best use your salon space. The following checklist will assist in organizing the decoration project.

1. Windows and drapes should be cleaned at least once a week.
2. Window displays should be changed regularly.
3. Make sure that the door to the salon is distinctive and clearly indicates the name of the salon.
4. Doors should be clean, easy to open, wide enough for wheelchair clients, and shatterproof if made of glass.
5. Clients should be furnished with a place to hang their coats, preferably a coat rack or open coat closet.
6. A special area should be provided for children in the side of the reception area.
7. Wall displays should be easy to clean and easy to change.
8. The reception desk should be well organized and well stocked with necessary items such as notepads, appointment cards, writing implements, price lists, and appointment books.
9. The reception area should contain comfortable chairs.
10. Walls within the styling area should be easy to clean.
11. Restrooms, mirrors, floors, and counter space around each work area should be kept clean.
12. Floors should be made of a nonporous substance that is long wearing and easy to clean.
13. Styling chairs should be comfortable and covered in an easy-to-clean, stain-resistant material.
14. A clean coffee pot and coffee cups should be part of the equipment in the styling area for the convenience of clients.
15. The exterior of the salon should be well maintained and well lit.

CHAPTER FIFTEEN SUMMARY

- A salon has a personality, dependent on original composition, management, operators, supplies and maintenance, and the work it produces. All parts must work well or else the salon will fall into trouble.
- To perform well, management must attend to all parts of the salon, help the staff succeed and participate, and develop management skills.
- Support systems include the bookkeeping system, supply room, supply system, working capital, receptionist, and maintenance department.

REVIEW QUESTIONS

1. What are the brains of the salon?
2. What is it called when employees work well together?
3. Who should a new, inexperienced operator work next to?
4. Who is called the "nerve center" of the salon?

Answers to Review Questions

CHAPTER ONE

1. Skin-care services are found in large, full-service salons and department store salons.
2. The home-neighborhood salon is the oldest type of salon existing today.
3. The financial structure is based on the owner's own personal financial security.
4. A franchise offers standardization.
5. The person who owns the most stock has the most control in an employee-owned corporation. Final decisions lie with those who hold the majority of the stock collectively.

CHAPTER TWO

1. A notary public must sign.
2. A deposit clause states that the landlord will hold your deposit to cover any damage not considered normal wear and tear.
3. A grocery store or drugstore might help your business.
4. Your lawyer should read the contract before you sign it.

CHAPTER THREE

1. The asbestos will have to be removed, at considerable expense.
2. A use tax is put on items purchased in another city and used by you to make a profit.
3. Liability insurance provides protection for losses resulting from legal liability.
4. Equipment and supply insurance covers damage, other than normal wear and tear, to everything in the salon.
5. The salon is required to withhold FICA taxes from an employee's wages.

CHAPTER FOUR

1. Leasing is a better option when you are cash-poor.
2. A bank would prefer to secure a loan with a house, car, stocks, bonds, or furniture.
3. Used equipment usually sells for 25 to 60 percent of its original value.
4. They combine the shampoo bowl and the styling station.

CHAPTER FIVE

1. The name of the salon should be on the door.
2. They should be changed at least once a month.
3. The receptionist should be responsible for watching children in the reception area.
4. The room will appear larger if painted white or a light color.
5. Shag carpets can catch people's heels, causing them to fall.

CHAPTER SIX

1. Stations have so much electrical equipment attached to them that they should be wired separately.
2. A styling chair should allow full comfort to the client while allowing the operator complete freedom of movement.
3. The dryer chairs should be the most comfortable.
4. They need ventilation because of the health hazards posed by some chemicals and materials used in nail services.
5. They will provide you with "loaners."

CHAPTER SEVEN

1. An inventory list is a sheet listing all the products on hand.
2. When they look cluttered, someone will straighten them out.
3. MSDS stands for "Material Safety Data Sheets."
4. The permanent wave is one of the most costly items.

CHAPTER EIGHT

1. The salon will spend more than $3,000.
2. The manager usually receives a straight salary.
3. A duty list assigns certain cleaning duties to each operator and employee.
4. Uniforms help maintain a standard look.
5. Survey forms should be passed out every three months.

CHAPTER NINE

1. ADA stands for "Americans with Disabilities Act."
2. Six conditions that might be included in the definition of disability are: obesity, suicidal tendencies, borderline personality disorders, traumatic stress syndrome, diabetes, and allergies to tobacco and chemicals.
3. Federal, state, and local governmental levels all have labor-related laws.

CHAPTER TEN

1. A percentage is a ratio of two figures.
2. "Each" price is the actual price on a unit of merchandise.
3. Salons pay 55–60 percent of retail price for goods they sell.
4. Profit on retail goods is usually 20–25 percent.
5. The major expense in a salon is wages.
6. Each operator could generate $20 per hour for haircuts.

CHAPTER ELEVEN

1. The report shows the operator's name and Social Security number and the totals for the month.
2. Employees are required to state the amount of tips over a specified figure on a form and return the form to you.
3. The most important record kept in a salon is the appointment book.

CHAPTER TWELVE

1. A five-day refresher course is recommended each year.
2. The officer is the school director or director of personnel.
3. You could get hiring information about other salons, price schedules, types of salons in the area, and management procedure information.

CHAPTER THIRTEEN

1. It should be run for three days in a row.
2. The first piece of information to record is how many calls came in from the ad.
3. Word-of-mouth is the most effective type of advertising.
4. The best time for a sale is when business is lowest during the year.
5. Each employee must take some responsibility for public relations.

CHAPTER FOURTEEN

1. Real profit is the amount of money left after all bills are paid.
2. Welcome Wagon greets new people in the community.
3. The person who does the selling should receive 15 percent commission.
4. Shades and fashions change so quickly that you don't want to be left with unsold stock.

CHAPTER FIFTEEN

1. Management is the brains of a salon.
2. It is called teamwork.
3. An inexperienced operator should work in the position next to an experienced operator.
4. The receptionist is the nerve center of the salon.

Index